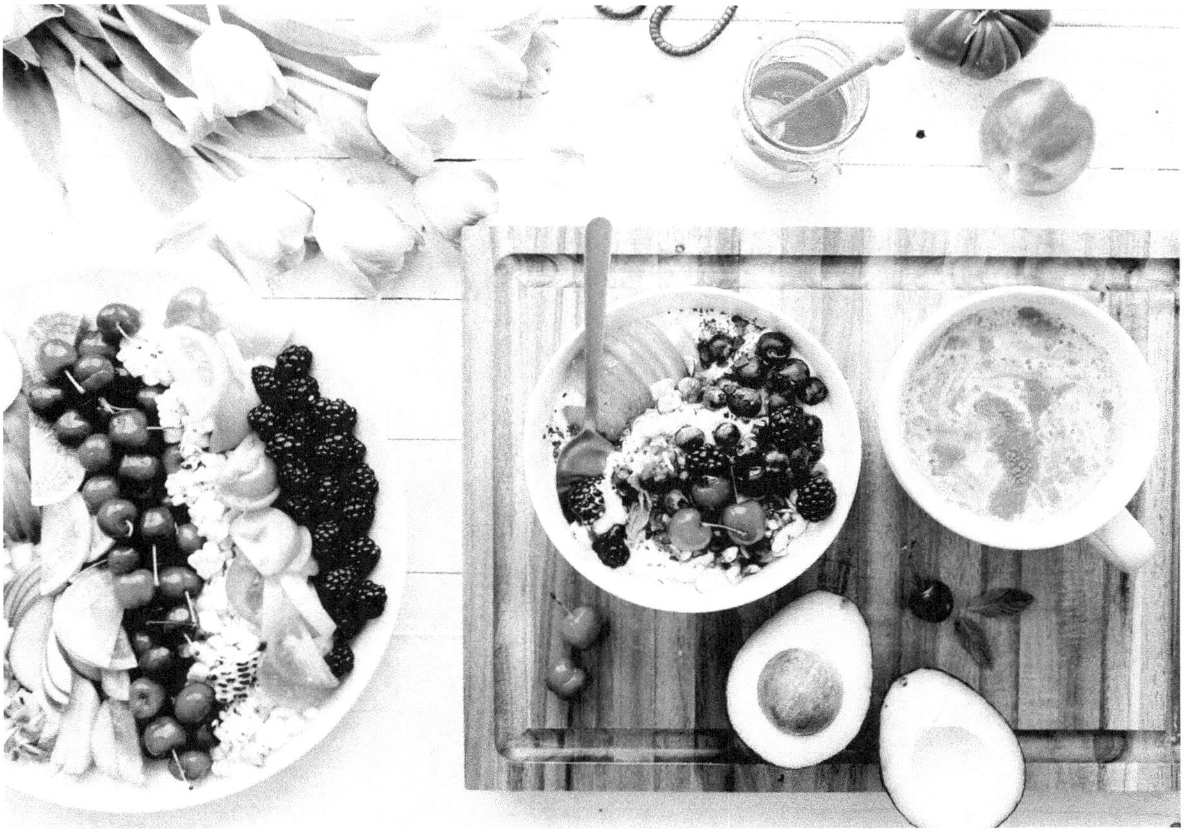

THE HEALTHY MEAL PREP COOKBOOK

101 Superfast and Easy Prep-and-Go Healthy Whole Food Recipes to Lose Weight and Heal Your Body

MICHELLE DORRANCE

© Copyright 2017 by Michelle Dorrance - All rights reserved.

This eBook is reproduced below with the goal of providing information that is as accurate and reliable as possible. Regardless, purchasing this eBook can be seen as consent to the fact that both the publisher and the author of this book are in no way experts on the topics discussed within and that any recommendations or suggestions that are made herein are for entertainment purposes only. Professionals should be consulted as needed before to undertaking any of the action endorsed herein.

This declaration is deemed fair and valid by both the American Bar Association and the Committee of Publishers Association and is legally binding throughout the United States.

Furthermore, the transmission, duplication or reproduction of any of the following work including specific information will be considered an illegal act irrespective of if it is done electronically or in print. This extends to creating a secondary or tertiary copy of the work or a recorded copy and is only allowed with an express written consent from the Publisher. All additional rights reserved.

The information in the following pages is broadly considered to be a truthful and accurate account of facts, and as such any inattention, use or misuse of the information in question by the reader will render any resulting actions solely under their purview. There are no scenarios in which the publisher or the original author of this work can be in any fashion deemed liable for any hardship or damages that may befall them after undertaking information described herein.

Additionally, the information in the following pages is intended only for informational purposes and should thus be thought of as universal. As befitting its nature, it is presented without assurance regarding its prolonged validity or interim quality. Trademarks that are mentioned are done without written consent and can in no way be considered an endorsement from the trademark holder.

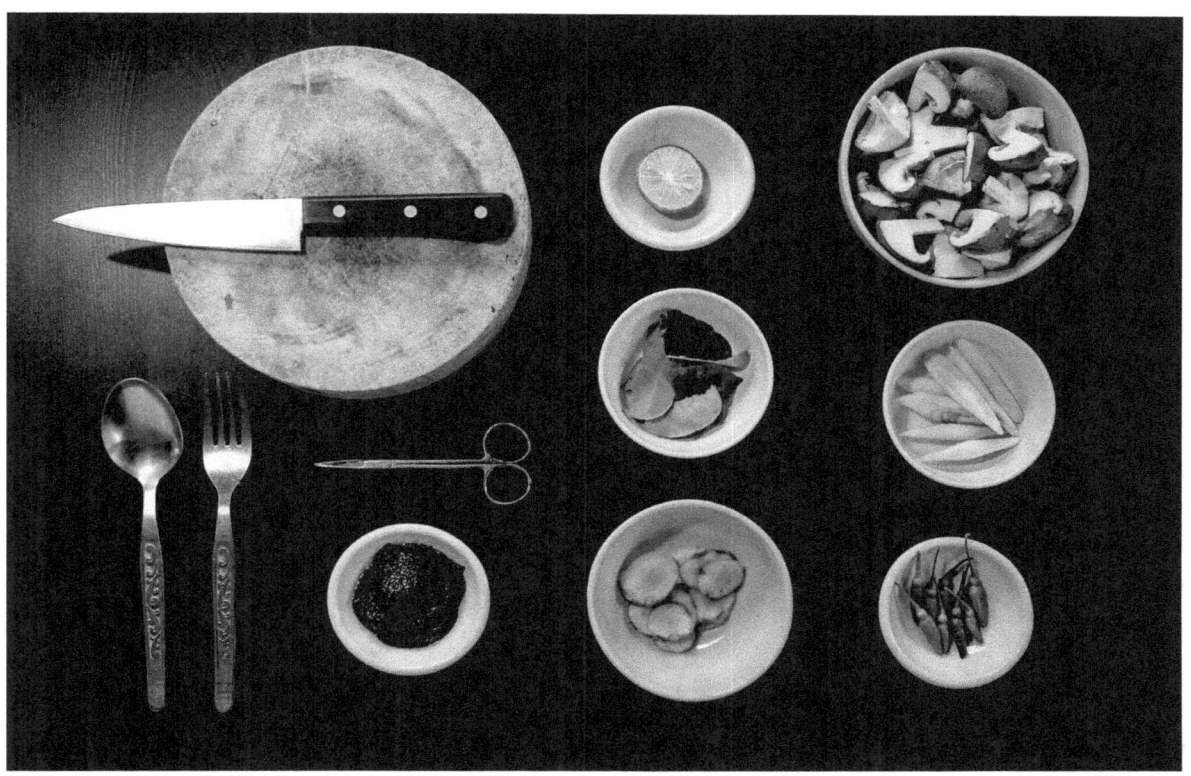

To all my Meal Prep fans, this book is dedicated to you. Without your loyalty and support, this book would never have been possible.

To my favorite taste-tasters – my husband, Todd, and my lovely girl Toma – thanks for trying all my cooking experiments (the good and the bad!) and for your love and throughout this amazing journey!

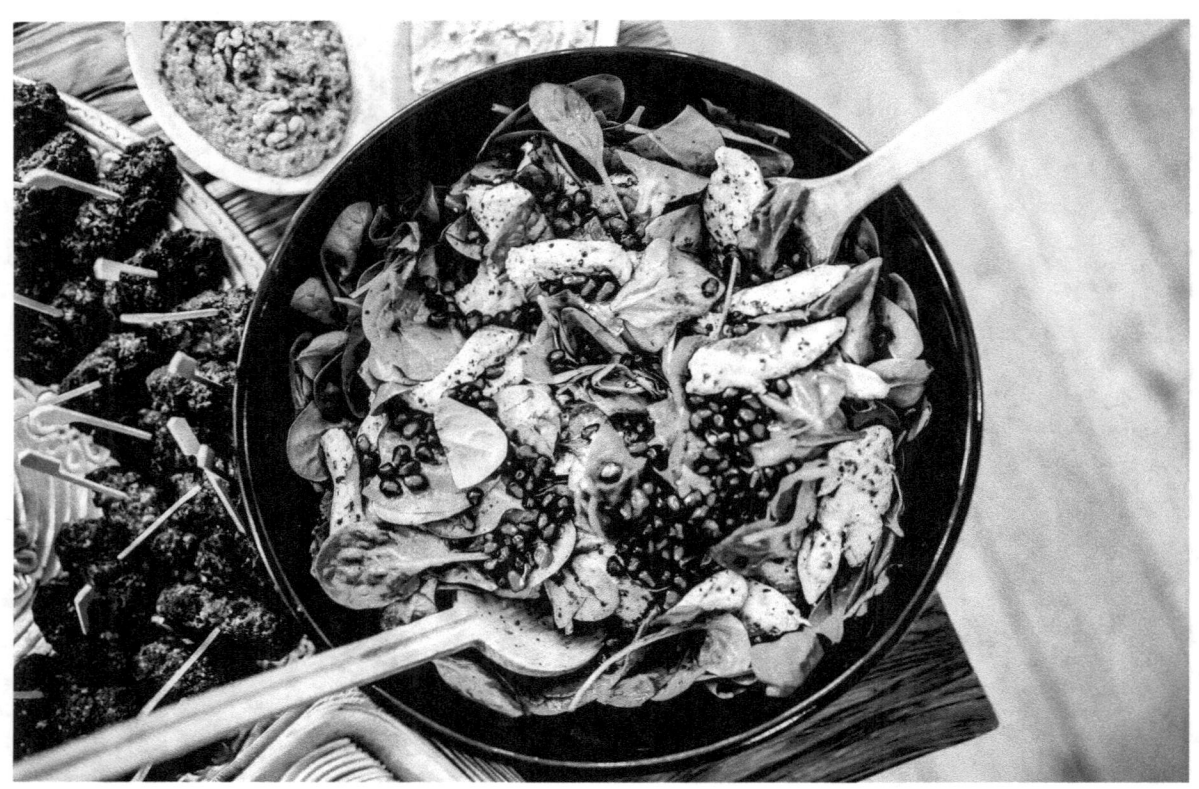

CONTENTS

Introduction 1
Chapter One: Meal Prep 3
    What is meal prepping? 3
    Why meal prep? 4
    Mistakes to avoid while meal prepping 4
Chapter Two: You are What You Eat 9
    Foods to enjoy 16
    Foods to minimize 18
    Foods to avoid 19
    Health information 20
Chapter Three: Beginning Your Meal Prep 23
    How to meal prep 23
    Kitchen equipment 24
    Money saving tips 26
    Food storage tips 27
Chapter Four: Storing Your Food 29
    7 Healthy freezer hacks 29
    Foods that do not freeze and Thaw well 32
    How to thaw foods safely? 33
    Meal Prep Sunday 36
    Measurement Conversions 38
    About The Recipes 39
Chapter Five: Recipes 41

Breakfast and smoothies 41

Soup and stew 64

Vegetarian Mains 92

Fish and seafood 116

Poultry 141

Meat 163

Salads and Vegetables 189

Snacks and Sides 210

Conclusion 231

Recipe Index 233

Introduction

Modern life is hectic. There's no escaping to this fact. And yet, we're supposed to work 8 hours a day (if we're lucky it's just 8 hours!) ferry kids to extracurricular activities, check on homework, attend meetings, concerts and events. And to top it off, we're supposed to eat well and exercise, too! I'm exhausted just thinking about it.

When I come home from work, everyone is hungry. "What's for dinner?" is the stock question. I used to not have an answer and hoped I could whip up something fabulous, healthy and great-tasting from the pantry without any forethought. Occasionally I would please everyone, but for the most part I was failing miserably. I'd think of something to make but not have a key ingredient. Or I'd have the ingredients but not the time it takes to prepare them. And forget about new recipes. Those were for weekends when I had the time and more energy to shop. I figured I needed a way to plan meals with my schedule in mind.

So, many years ago I came up with a way to plan meals with my busy schedule. Since then it has worked for me and I hope it can work for you, too!

As you explore the pages of this book, you'll not only realize that meal prep is the best way for you to stay on your diet and save money, but you'll also learn the step-by-step process on how to meal prep with your busy schedule and what you need to meal prep.
The last chapter of this book will contain the recipes that will foster a low carb, and gluten free diet.

The recipes I included in this book were carefully selected so they are easy to prepare, contain easy-to-find ingredients, keep nutrition in mind, and are delicious. Each recipes provides exact measurements for a serving size to help calories in check. A nutritional information is also available for each recipe, so you can make the healthiest decision for your individual needs.

With more than 115 dishes to choose from, you will find you really can save time, make meals more enjoyable, and eat healthier.

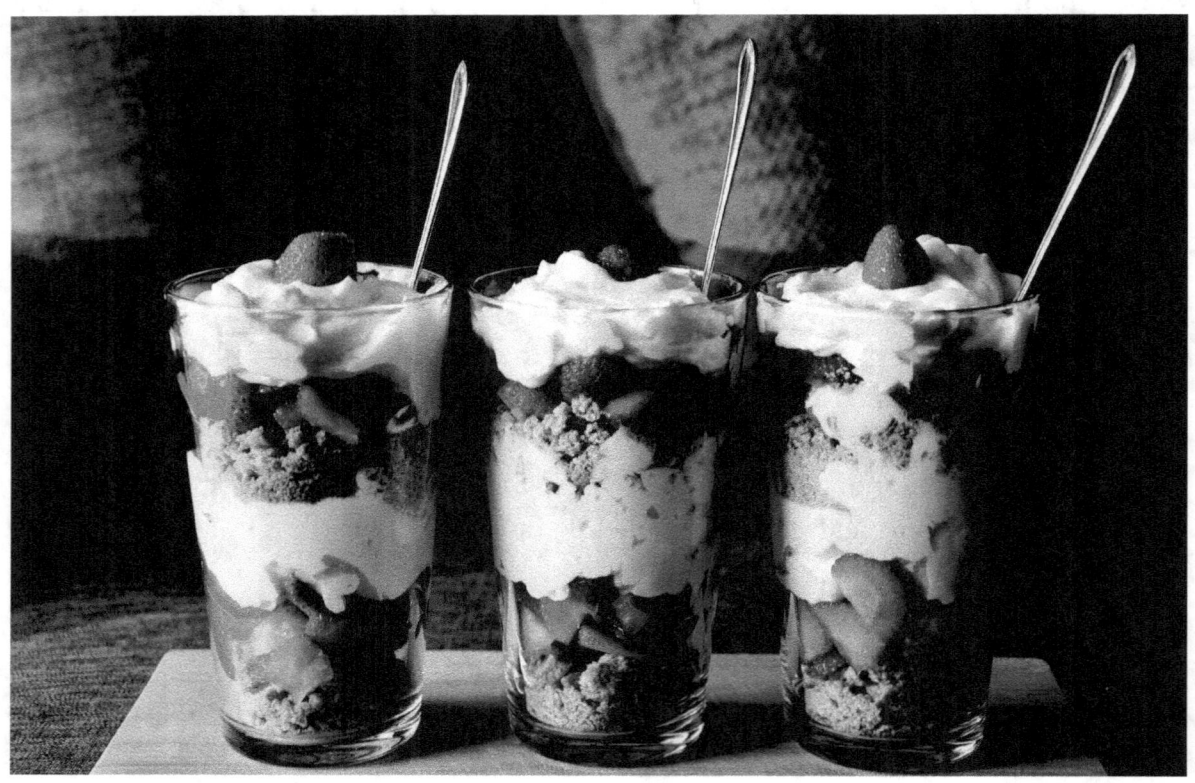

Let's get started!

Chapter One: Meal Prep

What is meal prepping?

Meal prep is defined as choosing a day to prepare your meals from start to finish. You will typically be making meals for longer than two days but less than four days. What you will be doing is planning the meal, cooking it, and packaging the meal and storing it in your fridge to be heated up and eaten at a later date.

Meal prep has taken off in the more recent years because it has been shown to help people maintain their diet. Meal prep comes in handy when you are a busy parent and don't have the time to be able to stand over a stove and cook a meal every night because you have to watch the kids or help with homework.

How long you plan to prep your meals is up to you. You may want to spend some hours in the kitchen preparing your meal for the next two to three days. If you are preparing meals for yourself, then it may only take you a few hours to do so. But if you are prepping food for the entire family, then you might be spending time more than you would when prepping only for yourself.

When prepping meal for the family, make an individual container for every member ensure that they get an everyone gets an even portion of the food that you are making. This is also going to help lower the stress of someone being upset because they did not get enough food, or they did not get something that was cooked since someone else took the last of what was made.

If you plan to do meals over four days, then you may want to consider freezing the meals so that they do not go bad and you don't lose food.

Why meal prep?

Why is it good to meal prep? Meal prep has a lot of advantages that most people do not know about, but, once they know about them, they will surely love it.

1. When you prep up to five days worth of meals, you'll be taking several hours out of a day; however, all of that time that you would be using during the week to cook these meals will be open for you to do something else. Not only are you going to be eliminating the time you have to spend cooking on a daily basis, but you are also going to be removing the time that you would have to wait for service at a restaurant.

2. Meal preparation saves you money! Obviously if you decide to eat out, you'll be spending more money than if you were to cook at home; however, cooking at home is not always going to be an option. Most of the meals that you can prep will cost you less than ten dollars a meal. So, think about how much you would typically spend on making sure that you have food in the house for everyone to eat. Now, figure out how much you would spend on eating out every day. Look at all of the money that you'll be saving.

3. Meal prepping will help you to stay on track so that you can keep your meals healthy.

Mistakes to avoid while meal prepping

When you are meal prepping, you are bound to make a few mistakes. You may make these mistakes even if you have mastered the basics of meal preparation. Sometimes, your problem will be that your food is soggy after it has been sitting in the fridge for a day or two and you feel like you should toss it out and find something that is a bit fresher.

When meal prep is done incorrectly, your food will tend to taste different and it is very likely that you would look for other foods that looks more appealing and fresher than what you have prepared. You sure want to avoid this costly mistake. Consider these:

1. Don't build a balanced meal. When you overeat one type of food, there is not going to be enough of another food in your diet, and it can end up screwing up your day. Take for example, if you are not getting enough carbohydrates because you are focusing too much on getting enough protein; then you'll begin to feel tired due to the fact that carbs are usually the source of energy. But, what if you are getting too many carbs but not enough protein? Then you'll discover that you are hungry well before it is time for you to eat dinner.

Dr. Jim White R.D.N says "Leaning heavily towards one macro can lead to deficiencies in other macros and other vital nutrients." For example, if you were to consume sixty percent protein, twenty percent fat, and twenty percent carbs you would be robbing yourself of B vitamins, fiber, and extra energy that you would generally get through a moderate carbohydrate diet.

The perfect macronutrient balance will be fifty percent carbs, thirty percent protein, and twenty percent fat. But, the ideal balance is going to depend on what your goal is going to end up being. Break down your macronutrients differently to ensure that you are getting what your body needs. You want to make sure that you are paying close attention to the nutritional breakdown of your macros too. And also, make sure that you don't forget to include fiber in your meal.

2. While it makes seem like you need to make all of your food in one day, you will be placing yourself in a position where you are most likely forget what

you have made and find something else to eat. Whenever you set cooked food in the fridge, it is typically going to go bad in three to five days; which is why you should try to prep a couple of times a week to make sure that the food that you are eating the next day tastes fresh.

Say you are prepping your food on Sunday, then the food that you have prepped is going to be good until Thursday. And, if you prep on Wednesday as well, then you'll be set for a few more days, and you won't have to worry about your food tasting terrible when you reheat it.

In the event that you want your food to last longer, prepare it and then freeze it to reduce the risk for foodborne illnesses. However, keep in mind that your food will not taste the same after it has been sitting in the freezer for several months.

3. Whenever you eat the same thing day in and day out, you'll get burned out on it quickly. So, you have to be smart about the food that you are preparing so that you are not eating the same thing every day. There has to be some wiggle room with the foods that you are making; just because you are eating healthy does not mean that you have to limit yourself to what you can eat.

Rather than steaming all of your vegetables, try roasting them or grilling them. There is a wide variety of carbohydrates too like sweet potatoes and quinoa that you can make for your meals as well.

When you are storing the food that you are prepping, store it in separate containers. All you have to do is take your vegetables and put them in separate bowls and do the same with all of the other food that you are making.

When you mix foods of different flavors in one container, it is very likely that the flavor of each food will change or all the foods will become soggy. So to avoid this, keep all of your food in separate containers.

4. If you are not keeping healthy food in your kitchen, then how do you expect to prepare healthy meals? Most of the time when you don't have a specific ingredient in your kitchen for a recipe you'll find it is easy to add in something that is not as nutritious. This is why you need to prep your meals beforehand and then make sure that you are stocking your kitchen accordingly.

It is a good idea to make sure that you are keeping your go-to ingredients on hand so that you have options for last minute meals in case one of your recipes falls through.

5. Meal prep is not complicated, but it will be if that is how you make it. You should not worry about complicated cooking methods that will cause you to spend hours over the stove. It is wise to cook things in bulk that way you are not spending too much time preparing.

You may also want to experiment with cooking styles to find a new way to enjoy your food. If you are a newbie in the kitchen, simplify things by using a crockpot where you can dump everything into it and let it cook for half a day. At the end of the time that it takes for it to prepare, you will have food that tastes as if you slaved over it, but you didn't.

Chapter Two: You are What You Eat

Some of the foods that are on the lists below will help you identify which foods are good to eat and which you cannot. It will also help you determine the foods you need to stick to and those you need to stay away from if you want to stick to a low-carb diet.

Essential Ingredients for Low-Carb Cooking

Fresh Herbs
1. Basil
2. Chives
3. Cilantro
4. Dill weed
5. Ginger root
6. Peppermint leaves
7. Thyme
8. Parsley
9. Rosemary

Shopping & storage tips

You are most likely going to want to try and purchase your fresh herbs from a farmer's market or from an organic store that is in your area. You have to be careful buying fresh herbs from a typical grocery store due to the fact that they are not always going to be fresh.

For the basil, parsley, and cilantro, you have to trim the ends and put them in a glass of water. There should only be about an inch of water in the glass that you are using. Make sure to use the herbs soon or else they will go bad because they are only going to stay fresh for a week. Do not refrigerate or else the leaves will turn black. You can also do this with any other long-stemmed herbs.

When you are dealing with herbs such as chives, rosemary, or thyme, you'll have to wrap them in plastic wrap and place them in the fridge. One of the compartments in the door will work for storage. Don't cover the herbs too tight, or the moisture that is trapped in the plastic will cause them to mold. Because of how they are stored, you'll not have to rinse the herbs before you use them. Throw them away when they begin to mold.

Cheese
1. Monterey Jack
2. Gruyere
3. Blue Cheese
4. Swiss cheese
5. Gouda
6. Cheddar
7. Munster
8. Fontina
9. Mozzarella

Shopping & storage tips
You can buy cheese in any grocery store. Make sure to grab the right cheese because there will be times where the wrong cheese is placed in the wrong space at the store. There is not going to be any indication that the cheese is low carb, so you'll have to go based off of the list.

Store the cheese in the fridge and used before it molds. You can also freeze the cheese. However, depending on the kind of cheese you have, the taste and texture may change especially if it has been stored in the freezer for several months.

Eggs
1. Deviled
2. Fried
3. Hard boiled
4. Poached
5. Scrambled
6. Soft-boiled

Shopping & storage tips

You can purchase eggs from the grocery store. However, it's better if you can get eggs fresh from a farm. If your eggs are from the store, place them in the fridge immediately because that is how you bought them. Farm fresh eggs can sit on your counter for a week before they go bad, but if you refrigerate them, they can stay good up to six months whereas store-bought eggs can last up to three months.

Dairy
1. Almond milk
2. Hemp milk

Shopping & storage tips

You are most likely will go to a health food store to get almond milk or hemp milk. Unless you are buying boxed milk, you'll have to put it in the fridge. Just like regular milk that you get from the store, it will have an expiration date. Almond milk is typically going to go bad after seven days while hemp milk will expire after ten days once you have opened it. In the event that you are buying shelf milk, it can sit on the shelf for several months unopened before it goes bad.

Fresh Produce
1. Cantaloupe
2. Peaches

3. Watermelon
4. Strawberry
5. Raspberry
6. Blackberries
7. Starfruit
8. Avocado

Shopping & storage tips

It's best to buy fresh produce in farmer's market because they sell locally grown produce. For the food not grown in your area, go to a grocery store. You need to make sure that you are checking your fruit because there may be mold on it and if there is mold on one, then all of the produce will be compromised. When it comes to storing your produce, place them on a paper towel in a single row so that they are not sitting on top of each other continually getting moisture dripped on them. You should produce in the fridge, make sure to place them on the crisper drawer. However, make sure that you are keeping your vegetables in one drawer and your fruit in the other so that the ethylene gas does not mix into your other foods and cause it to go bad before its time.

Frozen Produce
1. Squash
2. Spinach
3. Kale
4. Berries

Shopping & storage tips

Frozen produce are available in local grocery store. Try and grab the ones that are in the middle of the stack that way you are not getting the fruit that is thawed because the door is always being opened. The ones that are on the bottom will be the ones that are most likely going to be freezer burned. When you are storing your frozen produce, make sure that it is lying flat and does not have anything heavy placed on it once it goes in the freezer. If you set something substantial on it or you allow it to get bunched up in the corner of the freezer you'll be risking the bag being broken and the contents spilling everywhere, or freezer burn.

Meat, fish, poultry
1. Chicken (boneless and skinless)
2. Ground beef (85% lean or higher)
3. Ground turkey (93% lean or higher)
4. Salmon
5. Tilapia
6. Shrimp
7. Steak
8. Pork
9. Sausage
10. Tuna

Shopping & storage tips

If possible, purchase any meat that you get from a butcher because they usually get fish and meat in fresh every day and if they don't then they will know how to store it so that you are not going to be getting sick after you buy it. Your food needs to be stored in a container that is clean and can be sealed to create an airtight seal. Put it on the bottom shelf so that it is in the coldest part of the fridge and it is not leaking any of its juices onto your other foods in the event that something compromises the container. Don't eat meat that is past its expiration date. Most meat have a storage sticker on the bottom that will inform you of the best way to store that particular meat so that it will not contaminating your other foods.

Dried herbs & spices
1. Allspice
2. Anise seed

3. Annatto
4. Ground Basil
5. Cajun spices
6. Caraway
7. Caraway seeds
8. Cayenne
9. Chili powder
10. Chinese five spices

Shopping & storage tips

You can buy dried herbs and spices anywhere. There may be a spice shop in your area where you can get the spices that you want. When you are storing your herbs and spices, make sure that they are not in direct light or heat. You are most likely not going to want to keep them all in clear containers; but, there are some that will do better in a dark jar or tin.

Canned vegetables
1. Tuna
2. Salmon
3. Crab
4. Sardines
5. Tomatoes
6. Salsa
7. Pasta sauce (no sugar)
8. Tomato sauce (no sugar)
9. Green chilies
10. Tomato paste

Shopping & storage tips

You can purchase canned in grocery stores. When you are picking up the cans, make sure that there are no dents in the can or else the product inside can be compromised. When you get your cans home, don't allow them to sit in an area where they will be moisture or else they will rust. Whenever the rust is deep enough, there will be holes that are in the can or the lid and then there are going to be foodborne illnesses in the can compromising the food. Watch for can corrosion because the metal can cause the food to react chemically; especially with high acid food. And finally, do not allow your cans to come into contact with high temperatures.

Broth
1. Chicken bone broth
2. Turkey bone broth

Shopping & storage tips

Bone broth will be something that you'll have to make yourself. When it comes to storing the broth, strain it through a sieve and put the broth into ice cube trays before placing them in the freezer. From there you'll have to remove them from the ice trays and place it in a freezer proof container such as a stainless-steel dish.

Garlic
1. Clove

Shopping & storage tips

Garlic is available in local grocery store, farmers market, or a health food store. The garlic should be firm and should not contain any blemishes. To store it, get a brown paper bag and punch it full of air holes before placing your garlic in it and folding it over. When you do it this way, you'll be extending the life of your garlic. Make sure that you are placing the bag in a cool dark place. You don't need to use plastic bags, or they will accelerate the rate in which the garlic will spoil. And, don't put potatoes near your garlic because potatoes release gas that can spoil the garlic.

Cooking oils
1. Avocado oil
2. Coconut oil

Shopping & storage tips

Your grocery store will have all of the cooking oils that you will need to cook your food. Ensure that you are putting the cap back on the container whenever it is not being used. You should store all of your oils in a glass that is dark colored; so, if it comes in a plastic bottle, place it in a glass jar. Don't put your oil in an iron or copper container or else there will be a chemical reaction between the metal and the oil.

Foods to enjoy

Meat
- Meat that has been grass-fed
- Any fish that has been caught in the wild
- Pork and poultry that is pastured

Healthy Fats
Monounsaturated Fat
- Olive and Sesame oil
- Avocados
- Nuts (almonds, peanuts, macadamia, hazelnuts, and cashews)

Polyunsaturated Fat

- Omega threes that are often found in seafood or fatty fish
- Flaxseed
- Walnuts
- Soymilk

Vegetables
Greens
- Lettuce
- Bok choy
- Swiss chard
- Chives

Cruciferous vegetables
- Kale (the dark leaf one is the best for you)
- Radishes
- Kohlrabi

Other
- Summer squash
- Spaghetti squash
- Bamboo shoots
- Zucchini

Fruits
- Avocado
- Blueberries
- Apples
- Bananas
- Kiwis
- Papayas

Condiments and beverages
- Water (of course because it is one of the healthiest things that you can drink!)
- Tea (black tea and herbal tea are the best)
- Coffee (do not put creamer in it, though. If you cannot drink it black, then put cream or coconut milk in it for sweetness)
- Any spices or herbs
- Lime juice and zest
- Lemon juice and zest
- Foods that are fermented (kimchi, sauerkraut (make your own) and kombucha)
- Whey proteins
- Egg whites

Foods to minimize

Vegetables, fruits, mushrooms
- Red cabbage
- White cabbage
- Green cabbage
- Fennel
- Rutabaga
- Brussels sprouts

Animals and dairy
- Ghee
- Eggs
- Beef

Nuts and seeds
- Brazil nuts (however do not eat a lot of them because of the prominent level of selenium they contain)
- Hemp seeds
- Sunflower seeds

Soy products
- Soy sauce
- Natto
- Tempeh

Condiments
- Erythritol
- Swerve
- Stevia
- Arrowroot powder

Alcohol
- Unsweet spirits
- Dry white wine
- Dry red wine

Foods to avoid

Grains
- Wholemeal
- Corn
- Rye

Factory farmed fish and pork
- Fish that is high in mercury

- Fish inflamed with omega 6
- Fish with PCBs

Processed foods
- Food with carrageenan
- MSG
- BPAs
- Sulphites
- Artificial sweeteners

Beverages
- Soda (Regular or Diet) Drinking soda
- Wine Coolers
- Beer
- Lemonade and Fruit Juices
- Sweetened Teas
- Energy Drinks
- Sports Drinks
- Frappes and Other Frozen/Iced Coffees.

Health information

1. Protein

    Chicken, beef, and fish are excellent sources of protein. Try and aim for around 1.5 to 2.0 grams per kilogram of body weight. Or, go with 0.7 to 0.9 grams per pound.

2. Carbohydrates

Sweet potatoes, taro root, and even blueberries are sources of carbohydrates. There is some debate on how many carbs you should be intaking a day, but most doctors say that you need less than 125 grams.

3. Fruit

   Blackberries, avocados, and raspberries are just a few of the fruits that you can eat while you are on a low carb diet. Eat fifty grams of fruit a day.

4. Fat

   Chicken fat, goose fat, lard, and ghee will be some of the fats that you can eat on a low carb diet. Aim eating at least 22 grams of fat a day, but you may even want to go up to 36 grams depending on how many calories you are consuming.

5. Vegetables

   Bok choy, spinach, and chives are some of the best vegetables that you can eat on a low carb diet. Try and get at least 35 grams of vegetables a day. You may find that you will need more or less depending on how many calories you are consuming and how strict your diet is.

6. Total carbs vs. net carbs

Net carbs will be the total carbs that you will consume, but it is not going to include your fiber count in the total. If you are counting carbs for your diet, then you will have people informing you that there is a right way and a wrong way; however, this is not true. You need to count carbs the way that is best for you. There are plenty of methods that you will be able to follow online, or you can come up with your own way of counting.

Chapter Three: Beginning Your Meal Prep

How to meal prep

1. Start small.
   You don't want to overwhelm yourself by trying to start prepping too many meals at once. When you are just starting out, start with meals that you know how to cook and have perfected. Prep meals a few days at a time until you get the hang of it. The more that you prep, the more food you may end up wasting. Remember, the whole purpose behind meal prep is to save money, therefore, if food will go bad because you prepped too much, you are not going to be saving yourself any money.

2. Pick a day to meal prep.
   Since the food that you prep is only going to be good for a short period of time, make sure that you are picking two days to prepare your meals. Pick days that you will be able to dedicate a few hours in the kitchen so that you can get everything appropriately prepared. One example of the days that you could pick is Sundays and Thursdays because your meals that are made on Sunday are going to be good until Thursday. You can choose any days that you want, but think about how long things are going to stay right in the fridge before they mold or begin to taste funky.

3. Come up with meal prep ideas.
   Obviously, you need to have ideas of what you will cook. While you are first starting out, make sure you are sticking to the meals that you already know how to cook. However, as you begin to get the hang of it, you can branch out and start preparing other foods. Be mindful of how long it is going to be able to sit in the fridge as well as how it is going to taste after reheated.

4. Batch cook.

    Don't just cook a single meal at a time. If you are preparing chicken, then cook several pieces at once and place them in separate Tupperware containers. While this may seem like you are going to be eating the same thing every day, but that is far from the truth. You have the option of freezing food, so you can eat it later.

5. Be mindful of food safety.

    Don't eat raw meat! Make sure everything you cook is being cooked thoroughly or else you will end up making yourself sick. If you don't know how to cook something, then you'll need to check the package because it usually tells you what the internal temperature of the food. Whatever you store, your food it needs to be sealed tightly so that the food is not being compromised by bacteria.

Kitchen equipment

Having the right material will make your life so much easier because you are less likely to scramble around trying to find something that will work.

Must-Have

1. **A 6-quart slow cooker** that can be programmed. Having a slow cooker will be great for getting meals ready when you are busy with life. Having 6 quarts will ensure that you have enough to feed your family and then have leftovers. With the programmable option, you can set it to where it will cook for an extended period of time before it is put on warm so that your food is not cold.
2. **A hand blender** will be an excellent alternative to the countertop blender and can be used in making soups and sauces without any need to transfer the hot liquids. You can use it in your slow cooker.

3. **Sheets pans** will be a vital part of your meal prep. When you are cooking large batches of food, you can lay them down on the sheet and season them before cooking. This will ensure that you are able to get the seasoning to your food.
4. **A silicone baking mat** can be reusable and can be placed on your cookie sheets to keep your food from sticking to them.
5. **Glass storage containers** are perfect for storing your leftovers and prepping your meals since the lid is going to prevent leaks from happening. However, the glass container is easy to break. Keep that in mind to avoid accidents.
6. **Bento boxes** make meal prep easy because you can divide your items into separate slots to keep your food fresh instead of soaking in the juice of other foods.

Nice to have

1. **Mesh stainless steel strainers** will make the rinsing of your berries and vegetables more accessible. If you are eating rice or quinoa, you can rinse it as well without worrying about some of the grains slipping down into your drain.
2. **A canning funnel** will make filling mason jars more accessible so that you can portion your meals correctly without making a mess.
3. **16 oz. mason jars** will be perfect for meals and snacks that you prep because they can go directly into your fridge or freezer and with how tight the lid screws on, you'll have the peace of mind that you are not going to have to clean up any leaks.
4. **Baking cups** will be perfect for if you are making breakfast items. You'll not have to worry about anything getting stuck to the side of your muffin tin, and you will have the perfectly proportioned breakfast bite.
5. **Blenders** lets you create creamy dips or smoothies that help you get through your day without grabbing food from the vending machine.

6. If you want to, you are going to tenderize your meat before it is cooked so that it is not as robust. You can also use your **tenderizer** to inject the spices into the insides of the meat that you are cooking.

Money saving tips

1. **Plan ahead.**
   If you go into the store without a plan, then you will be buying whatever looks good, and that is not safe for your low carb diet. When you plan ahead, you are going to know what to get, and it is going to make your shopping trip more relaxed.

2. **Buy produce in season.**
   Whenever produce is bought in season, it is not only going to be good, but it is usually going to be cheap because it does not have to be shipped in from somewhere else.

3. **Buy and cook in bulk.**
   Whenever you buy in bulk, you'll be saving money because you won't have to buy several packages of the same meat at different prices. And, whatever you don't eat, or cook can be put in the freezer.

4. **Buy the largest package.**
   Buying in bulk does not mean that you have to buy the biggest package that is on the shelf. It means that you purchase the package that has the most in it so that you are able to get the most out of the meat or vegetables that you are preparing.

5. **Use sales and coupons.**
   Sometimes stores put their meat and various other products on sale to get rid of the extra that is on their shelf or to get rid of the meat before it expires.

As long as you plan on cooking it soon, you'll not have to worry about getting sick. And, you'll be able to find coupons online and even in the Sunday paper. The voucher may not be for a lot of money off, but a little bit of money over time is going to add up in the long run. And, you will be glad that you have those coupons when you are running low on money.

Food storage tips

1. **Organize your refrigerator, freezer, and pantry.**
   Get rid of the food, condiments, or beverages that you don't use by either throwing them away or giving them out to those you think might need it. Once you have gotten rid of everything that is not going to benefit you, make sure that anything left is placed in the fridge to where it is not stacked and causing other things to leak or break. Once a seal is broken, it is going to compromise the food, and you don't want to risk eating it because you are going to end up getting sick. For your pantry, make sure that you group everything together so that it is easier for you to find.

2. **Label your containers**.
   If you are canning your food, then make sure that you are labeling what is in it, and the date. You can do this with any Tupperware that you are putting in the fridge.

3. **Consider expiration dates.**
   When something has an expiration date that is getting close, you put it at the front of the fridge or the pantry so that you are grabbing it first rather than grabbing something that will be able to sit there for a little while longer.

4. **Clean daily.**
   Make sure you throw things away that are bad. The less mold that is in your fridge, the less likely your food is to be compromised by bacteria.

Chapter Four: Storing Your Food

7 Healthy freezer hacks

1. **Wrap in freezer paper and label**

    a. Buy your meat.

    The fresher the meat, the better it will freeze and the less likely it will have a funny taste whenever it is thawed and cooked.

    b. Get rid of the original packaging.

    You can freeze the food in the regular packaging, but you may not want to because it will be permeable to air and that will give your meat to get freezer burned.

    c. Get rid of any excess fat as well any bones that may cut the wrapper and cause your meat to become compromised.

    d. Lay out a sheet of your freezer wrap on a clean surface. Make sure that you are using a piece that is large enough to wrap the meat up three times.

    e. Make sure you are placing a piece of paper between the meats so that you don't have to unthaw the entire package if you are not ready to eat all of it.

2. **Keep greens on reserve.**

Greens are always healthy. The good thing about greens is that you can always add them in your recipes if you want. Make sure that you are keeping your greens in your crisper drawer. But remember, don't let your greens stay in the fridge for too long or else they will go bad. When your veggies go bad, it release gas that may negatively affect other veggies as well.

2. **Reusable shopping bags.**

Whenever you go to the grocery store, and you get the plastic bags, you'll be contributing to the landfills becoming overfilled. This is why you need to buy reusable bags. Reusable bags are way stronger than plastic bags anyway. Not just that, they can also store products much more than plastic bags can do.

3. **Vacuum-seal everything.**

When you vacuum seal your food, you'll be taking the air out of it so that it can stay fresh longer. You'll have the option of going to the store and buy a vacuum sealer, or you can use a straw and Ziploc bags. When you are using a straw, you will need to seal most of the bag but leave enough room for the straw to be placed in the bag. Once it has been sealed, suck all of the air out of the bag and then quickly pull the straw out of the bag and finish sealing it.

4. **Save burning food.**

There will be ways that you can save food from freezer burn and here is how:

   a. Chill food before you freeze it. Take your warm food and place it in an ice bath allowing the temperature to drop slowly so that your food freezes more efficiently.
   b. Use a thermometer to measure the temperature of the food that is in your freezer. Keep in mind that if you take the food out of the freezer multiple times, you'll be placing it at a higher risk for freezer burn.
   c. If you want to freeze your food correctly, keep your freezer at 0 degrees F or below because anything above that will cause the food to deteriorate at a faster rate.

5. **Freeze fresh herbs**

    a. Know that most of the herbs that you freeze are not going to taste the same once you thaw them.

    b. Collect your herbs once you have washed them and drained all of the excess water off of them.

    c. Ensure that there is no dirt left on the herbs after they have been washed. Leaving soil on them is going to cause their taste to change as well.

    d. Place foil or parchment paper on a tray.

    e. Place the herbs on the shelf and place in the freezer.

    f. Once frozen they can be removed from the freezer and placed in a freezer container that is going to hold all of your herbs. Make sure that you put a date on the herbs because they will go bad in two months.

6. **Blanch vegetables before freezing.**

Blanching is the process in which you will take your plants and boil them until they are partly cooked. This will save your vegetables that you are freezing so that they don't have colors or textures that are off. It will also help to preserve the flavor so that when it is thawed out, the vegetables would not taste bland.

    a. The first thing you'll need to do is boil your water while you clean your vegetables.

    b. Next, you'll put your vegetables in your pot and allow them to cook for a certain amount of time. The time will depend on the vegetable that you are blanching.

c. Once your vegetables have been blanched, drain them and put them into an ice bath instantly so that the cooking process is stopped, and your vegetables don't continue to become overcooked.
   d. After you have cooled the vegetables down, drain it once more and try and get all of the liquid out of them. The more liquid that is in the vegetable, the more inferior the quality of the food will be.
   e. Now place your vegetables in a freezer bag and put it in the freezer.

There are some vegetables that do not have to be blanched to be frozen such as corn and tomatoes.

Foods that do not freeze and Thaw well

Vegetables: Cabbage, Cucumbers, lettuce, onions, bell peppers, potatoes, radishes, garlic, onion, and sprouts.

Fruits: Apples, citrus, fruits, grapes, and melons

Dairy: Soft cheeses, cottage cheese, cream cheese, custard, and cream

Other: Canned food still in cans, eggs in shells, fried foods, pastas cooked beyond al dente.

Milk sauces: It will become curdled and separate.

Curry: A musty odor will occur as it freezes.

(Note: Some of these ingredients will freeze well within a recipe. However, the texture may change if frozen as a single ingredient.)

How to thaw foods safely?

1. Thawing meat, poultry, fish & seafood.
Do not allow your meat to sit out at room temperature for more than two hours.

Fridge thawing

You'll have to make sure that you plan the meal ahead of time so that you can allow the meat to thaw thoroughly. It will usually require twenty-four hours for every five pounds. Even the smaller pound sized meats will take at least twenty-four hours. Whenever you are using the refrigerator, keep these things in mind.

   a. Freeze your items on a plate or in a bowl to prevent leaking.
   b. There will be parts of your fridge that keep your food colder than others.
   c. Food will take longer to thaw if your fridge is set to a lower temperature.

Once your meat is thawed, make sure to use your meat within a day or two because most food go bad after that. Some red meats though can stay safe for three days. When meat is thawed in a fridge, it can be refrozen without having to be cooked, but don't be surprised if the taste of the food changes.

Cold water

This will be a faster strategy and will require you to pay close attention to the meat. Ensure that it is in a leak-proof package so that the environments bacteria cannot get into the food. Meat usually absorbs water as well, and you are not going to want that because it will produce a product that is watery and does not taste right.

You should keep the bag in cold water for up to three hours depending on how much you are trying to thaw. Make sure you are checking it and changing the water every thirty minutes to ensure it defrosts thoroughly.

You'll need to cook the food once it is fully thawed. If you plan on refreezing it, you'll have to prepare the food first.

Microwave thawing

This will be the riskiest way to thaw meat because it will thaw unevenly. This is not the recommended way to thaw food, but it will work if you are in a hurry. Make sure that you are cooking your meat as soon as it is thawed because it is being warmed up and entering a dangerous temperature. If you wait for your food to cook, you will risk bacteria getting into your food and causing the food to rot. If you will freeze your food again, make sure you are cooking it beforehand.

2. Thawing prepared dishes

Refrigerator thaw

This will be the most extended method once again, but it will be the best way for you to ensure you are preserving your food quality. And, if you don't eat the meal, you will be able to place it right back into the freezer without worrying about the food being compromised.

Cold water

You can wrap your meal in a freezer bag and place it in the cold water as you did earlier. You'll need to change out the water every thirty minutes so that the water does not leak into the food. You should use this method whenever possible because it will be the safest way for your food to be thawed.

The downside is that you cannot refreeze the food once you have used this method.

3. **Thawing vegetables & fruits**

The safest way to thaw vegetables and fruits is to use cold water because it will save the flavor for your food as well as making sure that you are not heating the produce up too much and compromising it. It is only going to take around ten minutes for the vegetables or fruit to be thawed out. Ensure you are squeezing out excess water before you cook it or else it will be water and not taste right.

You also need to inspect your vegetables and fruits to see if they accidentally thawed in the freezer which can be measured by looking for ice crystals. If they still contain ice crystals, they can be refrozen, but the taste and texture will probably end up changing.

4. **What not to do**

- When thawing meat, don't use hot water because you will be changing the internal temperature of the meat and it will be put at risk for bacteria growing on it.
- Don't leave out on the counter because the exposure to the room temperature will make it to where the rotting process is activated.
- Don't allow food to be refrozen after it has been thawed in the sink or the microwave unless you cook it first.
- Don't allow to thaw outside of the packaging because exposure to air will cause the food to become spoiled or harden.
- Don't try and refreeze food that has already thawed in the freezer.
- Don't freeze meat that has expired.

Meal Prep Sunday

Step 1: Check your calendar.

Make sure you are looking at the days in between when you are preparing your meals. Like I said earlier, try and meal prep at least two days a week, but of course, you can meal prep for an entire week. Just make sure you are considering how long things can sit in the fridge and stay good before they start to turn bad.

Step 2: Make a menu.

Having a list of which you'll follow for the week or for the two weeks. Having a menu will help you when it comes to cooking your food so that you don't have to try and think of something to make for that day. It also helps your family know what is for dinner or lunch the next day. You may even want to get a board and put that week's menu on the board, so everyone can see it.

Step 3: Go food shopping.

Get only the food that is on your menu. This will assist you in making sure that you are not getting something that is not going to help your diet. Plus, as you saw earlier, it will make your shopping trip faster.

Step 4: Prep & pack your food

    a. Prep your ingredients
        — Proteins: Your meat will need to be thoroughly cooked. When handling raw meat, wash your hands and the utensils that you will use.
        — Produce: Blanch or roast your vegetables depending on how you want them to be cooked. You can also eat them raw, but they need to be washed to get rid of any dirt or pesticides.

— Grains: Any grains need to be cooked. When cooking grains, make sure not to cook other products with it, i.e., do not cook rice with quinoa. You can prepare things like oatmeal and not cook it, but keep it away from anything else you are making.

b. Store smart.
It is a good idea to keep everything in separate containers when putting it in the fridge. This way your flavors are not mixing together and causing your food to taste different than if you were to eat it right after you cooked it.

c. Pack up to-go meals
once you are ready to, put all of your microwave items together to ensure you can microwave them. Other non-microwavable foods should be in a separate container.

Measurement Conversions

Use it for accurate measuring of the necessary ingredients.

Measurement Conversion Chart

Cup	Fluid Ounces	Tablespoons	Teaspoons	Milliliters
1 cup	8 oz	16 tbsp	48 tsp	237 ml
¾ cup	6 oz	12 tbsp	36 tsp	177 ml
⅔ cup	5 oz	11 tbsp	32 tsp	158 ml
½ cup	4 oz	8 tbsp	24 tsp	118 ml
⅓ c	3 oz	5 tbsp	16 tsp	79 ml
¼ c	2 oz	4 tbsp	12 tsp	59 ml
⅛ c	1 oz	2 tbsp	6 tsp	30 ml
1/16 c	½ oz	1 tbsp	3 tsp	15 ml

Measurements Conversions

1 c	=	½ pint
2 cups	=	1 pint
4 cups	=	1 quart
2 pints	=	1 quart
4 quarts	=	1 gallon
8 quarts	=	1 peck
4 pecks	=	1 bushel
3 tsp	=	1 tablespoon
4 tbsp	=	¼ cup
5 ⅓ tbsp	=	⅓ cup
8 tbsp	=	½ cup

Safe Meat Temperatures Cooking Times

Beef ...140°F... rare ... safe to eat
Beef ...160°F ... medium ... safe to eat
Beef ...170°F ... well-done ... safe to eat
Pork roast ... 165°F ... done ...safe to eat
Lamb roast ... 145°F ...safe to eat
Pork or Lamb, ground ...160°F ...safe to eat
Ham, precooked ... 140°F ... done
Chicken, whole ... 180°F ... safe to eat
Turkey, whole... 180°F... in thick part of thigh
Stuffing in poultry ... 165°F ... safe to eat

Oven Temperature Conversion Chart

Very low	250 - 275°F =	121 - 135°C
Slow Cook	300 - 325°F =	149 - 163°C
Moderate Heat	350 - 375°F =	177 - 191°C
High Heat	400 - 425°F =	204 - 218°C
Very Hot	450 - 475°F =	232 - 246°C
Extremely Hot	500 - 252°F =	260 - 274 °C

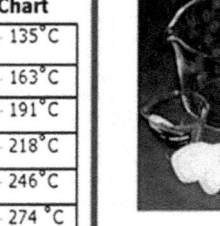

About The Recipes

The recipes in this book were chosen for appeal, ease of preparation, and speed.

With very few exceptions, you'll be ready in 30 minutes or less, start to finish. And almost every recipes requires no more than eight everyday ingredients to prepare.
All recipes include nutritional information, and also strategies for planning, shopping, prepping, cooking, storing, and freezing, including instructions for serving and reheating, so you can choose to eat the dishes straightaway or save them for another time.

Each recipe had a set upper limit on the amount of fat and sodium – no more than 35 percent of calories from fat and no more than 140 milligrams of sodium per serving.

Let's cook!

Chapter Five: Recipes

Breakfast and smoothies

1. Asparagus with browned butter and creamy eggs

(Serves: 2 / **Prep time:** 10 minutes / **Cooking time:** 15 minutes)

Nutritional Information (Per Serving)
Calories: 1080
Carbs: 19 g
Protein: 39 g
Fat: 96 g
Fiber: 1 g
Sodium: 5 mg

Ingredients
- Butter (5 ounces)
- Eggs (4)
- Lemon juice (1 ½ tablespoons)
- Cheese of your choice (3 ounces, grated)
- Olive oil (1 tablespoon)
- Sour cream (8 tablespoons)
- Asparagus (1 ½ pounds)
- Cayenne pepper (to taste)

Instructions
1. Melt the butter and add eggs into your scramble. Don't overcook the eggs.

2. Remove the eggs from the pan and put it in a blender, mix in cheese and sour cream. You should blend until it becomes creamy. Then add seasonings.
3. Roast your asparagus in olive oil, season and set aside.
4. Sauté 3 ounces of butter in a pan until golden brown. Allow to cool and add lemon juice.
5. Place asparagus in frying pan and stir with roasted butter.
6. Serve with sautéed butter and eggs.

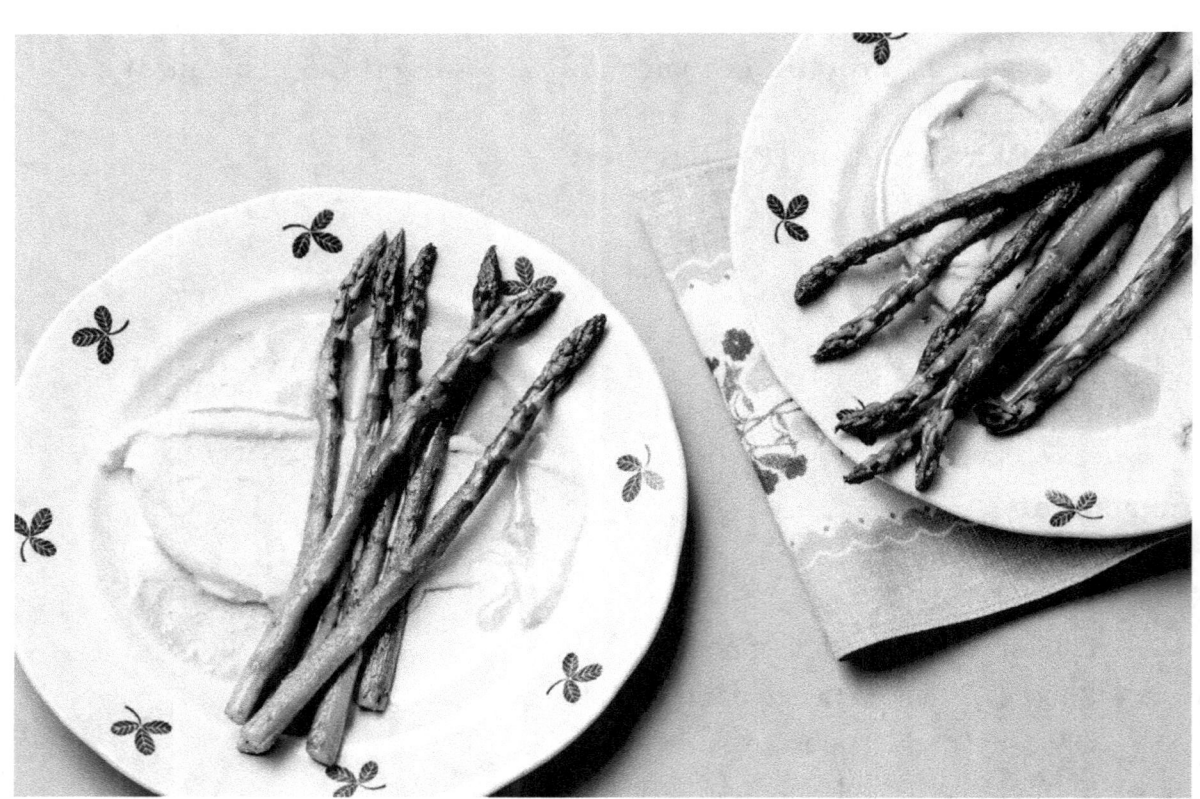

(**Freezer:** 3 months / **Microwave:** 1 ½ minutes)

2. Bacon Hash

(**Serves**: 2 / **Prep time:** 10 minutes / **Cooking time:** 15 minutes)

Nutritional Information (Per Serving)
Calories: 366
Carbs: 11 g
Protein: 23 g
Fat: 24 g
Fiber: 2 g
Sodium: 7.1 mg

Ingredients
- Eggs (4)
- Pepper (1)
- Bacon (6 slices)
- Onion (1)
- Jalapeno (optional)

Instructions
1. Cut the onion and pepper into thin slices.
2. Dice up the jalapeno.
3. Fry in a cast iron skillet.
4. Remove and chop the bacon in the food processor.
5. Mix everything together.
6. Cook hash until bacon is crisp.

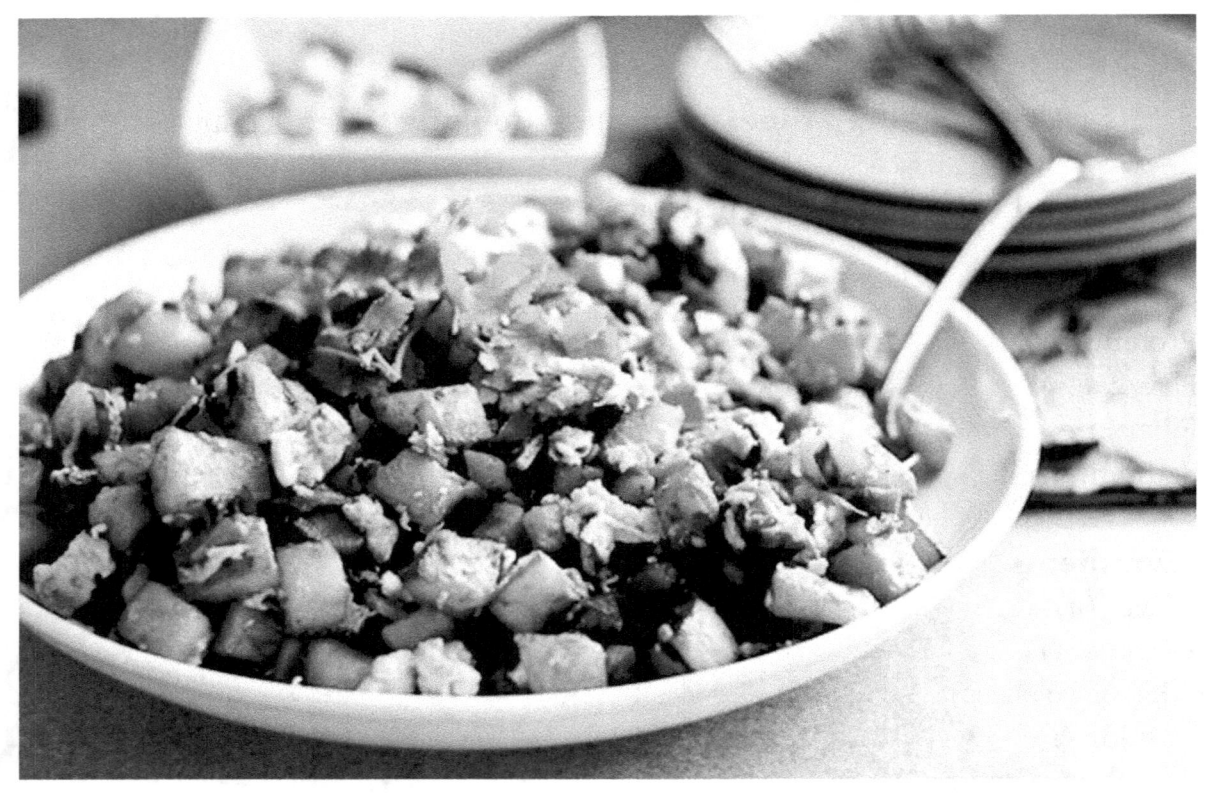

(**Freezer:** 2 months / **Microwave:** 2 minutes)

3. Inside Out Scotch Eggs

(**Serves:** 12 eggs / **Prep time:** 5 minutes / **Cooking time:** 20 minutes)

Nutritional Information (Per Serving)
Calories 168
Carbohydrates 0.25 g
Protein 12 g
Fiber: 20 g
Sodium 2 mg

Ingredients
- Avocado (optional)
- Eggs (12)
- Ground sausage (12 ounces)

Instructions
1. Divide your sausage up into one-ounce portions.
2. Place into a muffin tin so that it is about half an inch thick.
3. Put an egg in each cup.
4. Cook at 350 degrees oven for about twenty minutes.
5. Remove from the oven and enjoy with avocado if you desire to.

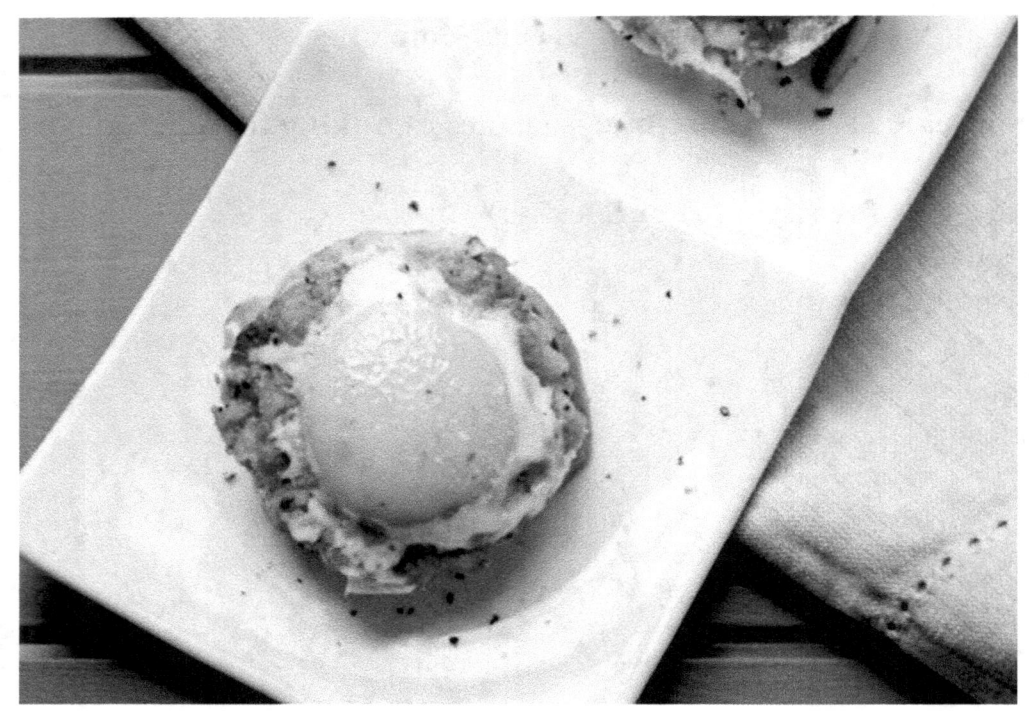

(**Freezer:** 1 week / **Microwave:** 1 ½ minutes)

4. Low carb Starbucks pink drink

(**Serves:** 4 / **Prep time:** 5 minutes / **Cooking time:** 25 minutes)

Nutritional Information (Per Serving)
Calories: 129
Carbs: 7 g
Protein: 2 g
Fat; 3 g
Fiber: 1.5 g
Sodium: 0 mg

Ingredients
- Ice (handful)
- Acai green tea (4 bags)
- Strawberries (2 cups, fresh)
- Hibiscus tea (4 packs)
- Coconut milk (1 ½ cup)
- Boiling water (2 cups)
- Erythritol (1/4 cup)

Instructions
1. Make the tea in a jar with the boiling water.
2. Take the tea bags out and mix in the sweetener so that it fully dissolves. Allow the tea to cool.
3. Place the cold tea and the strawberries in your blender and blend until completely smooth.

(**Freezer:** none / **Microwave:** none)

5. Breakfast stuffed peppers

(**Serves:** 4 / **Prep time:** 15 minutes / **Cooking time:** 50 minutes)

Nutritional Information (Per Serving)
Calories: 307
Carbs: 41 g
Protein: 13 g
Fat: 17 g
Fiber: 3.3 g
Sodium: 357 mg

Ingredients
- Bell peppers (4, halved, cored, seeded)
- Cooking fat (1 tablespoon)
- Eggs (8, beaten)
- Bacon (6 slices)
- Mushrooms (1 cup, sliced)
- Garlic powder (1/2 teaspoons)
- Onion (1, diced)
- Tomato (1, diced)
- Baby spinach (3 cups)

Instructions
1. Turn the oven on to 375 F.
2. Melt the fat.
3. Sauté the onions for around four minutes
4. Toss in tomatoes and mushrooms for another two minutes.
5. Next, add the spinach and cook until wilted.
6. Season to taste.
7. Divide and put into the bell peppers.
8. Finish off with egg mix and bacon.

9. Cook for forty minutes in the oven.

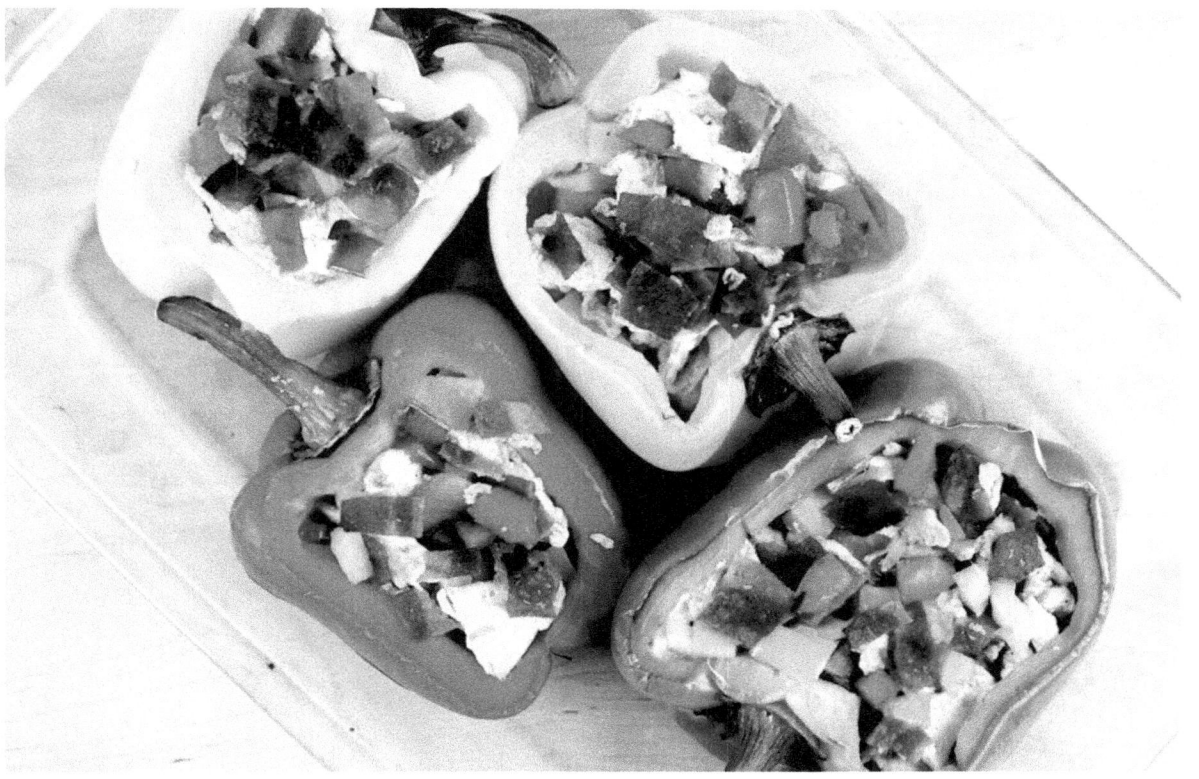

(**Freezer:** 1 month / **Microwave:** 3 minutes)

6. Radish scramble

(**Serves:** 2 / **Prep time:** 5 minutes / **Cooking time:** 21 minutes)

Nutritional Information (Per Serving)
Calories: 777
Carbs: 5 g
Protein: 64 g
Fat: 55 g
Fiber: 1 g
Sodium: 862 mg

Ingredients
- Pepper (to taste)
- Flank steak (8 ounces)
- Eggs (4)
- Radishes (6 ounces)
- Cheddar cheese (4 ounces)
- Cubetti pancetta (2 ounces)

Instructions
1. Preheat the oven to 450 degrees.
2. Pan fry the flank steak.
3. Wash radishes and quarter.
4. Pan fry radishes and pancetta. Radishes need to be golden brown.
5. Slice the flank steak and add into the pan.
6. Break the eggs and cover in cheese.
7. Season to taste and cook for a minute.
8. Move to the oven and bake for eight minutes.
9. Broil for an additional four minutes.

(**Freezer:** 2 months / **Microwave:** 2 minutes)

7. Green smoothie

(**Serves:** 1 / **Prep time:** 10 minutes / **Cooking time:** none)

Nutritional Information (Per Serving)
Calories: 184.2
Protein: 4.3 g
Fat: 1.3 g
Carbs: 44.6 g
Fiber: 5.4 g
Sodium: 87 mg

Ingredients
- Ice (handful)
- Water (1 cup)
- Banana (1/2)
- Lemon juice (1 cup)
- Kale (2 sticks, remove stems)
- Ginger (a slice, fresh, peeled)
- Spinach (2 handfuls)
- Cucumber (1/2 peeled)
- Parsley (handful, fresh)

Instructions
1. Put everything into a blender.
2. Blend until smooth.
3. Enjoy!

(**Freezer:** none / **Microwave:** none)

8. Spaghetti squash pancakes

(**Serves:** 2 / **Prep time:** 5 minutes / **Cooking time:** 15 minutes)

Nutritional Information (Per Serving)
Calories: 287
Carbs: 10 grams
Protein: 19 grams
Fat: 18 grams
Fiber: 3.3 g
Sodium: 1,219.2 mg

Ingredients
- Parmesan cheese (1 ounce)
- Bacon (4 slices)
- Onion powder (1 teaspoon)
- Eggs (2)
- Pepper (1 teaspoon)
- Spaghetti squash (10 ounces, cooked)
- (1 teaspoon)
- Garlic powder (1 teaspoon)

Instructions
1. Prepare your squash.
2. Cook the bacon until it reaches your desired crispiness.
3. Add the eggs, spices, cheese, and squash in a bowl and mix together
4. Crumble bacon into the pot.
5. Heat up the grease from the bacon.
6. Add the mix into the fat into four piles.
7. Cook until the bottom browns and batter slightly boils, then flip.
8. You may serve with some sour cream or chives.

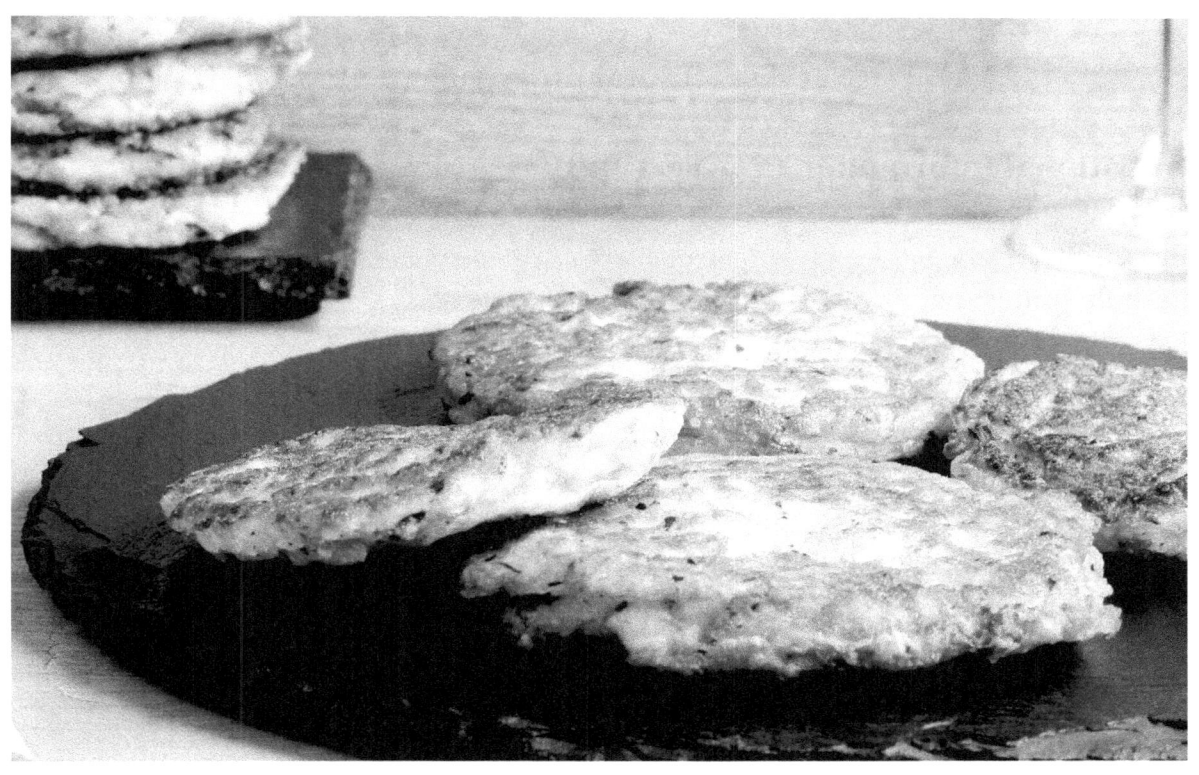

(**Freezer:** 2 months / **Microwave:** 1 ½ minutes)

9. Keto Iced Coffee

(Serves: 1 / **Total time:** 5 minutes)

Nutritional Information (Per Serving)
Calories: 340
Protein: 0 g
Carbohydrates: 0g
Fat: 38g
Fiber: 0 g
Sodium: 0 mg

Ingredients
- Ice cubes (a handful)
- Ground coffee (2 tablespoons, make sure it is a coarse ground so that it does not fall through your coffee filter)
- Boiling water (1 cup)
- Keto condensed milk (2 tablespoons or to taste)

Instructions
1. Pour your Keto condensed milk into a glass.
2. Place your coffee in the filter. Make sure that the coffee is evened out in the screen before you place it on top of the glass.
3. Dump around two tablespoons of water into your filter so that the coffee has a chance to begin to swell. Pour the rest of the liquid into the screen.
4. Cover the filter with some kind of lid and allow it to drip into the cup for around five minutes.

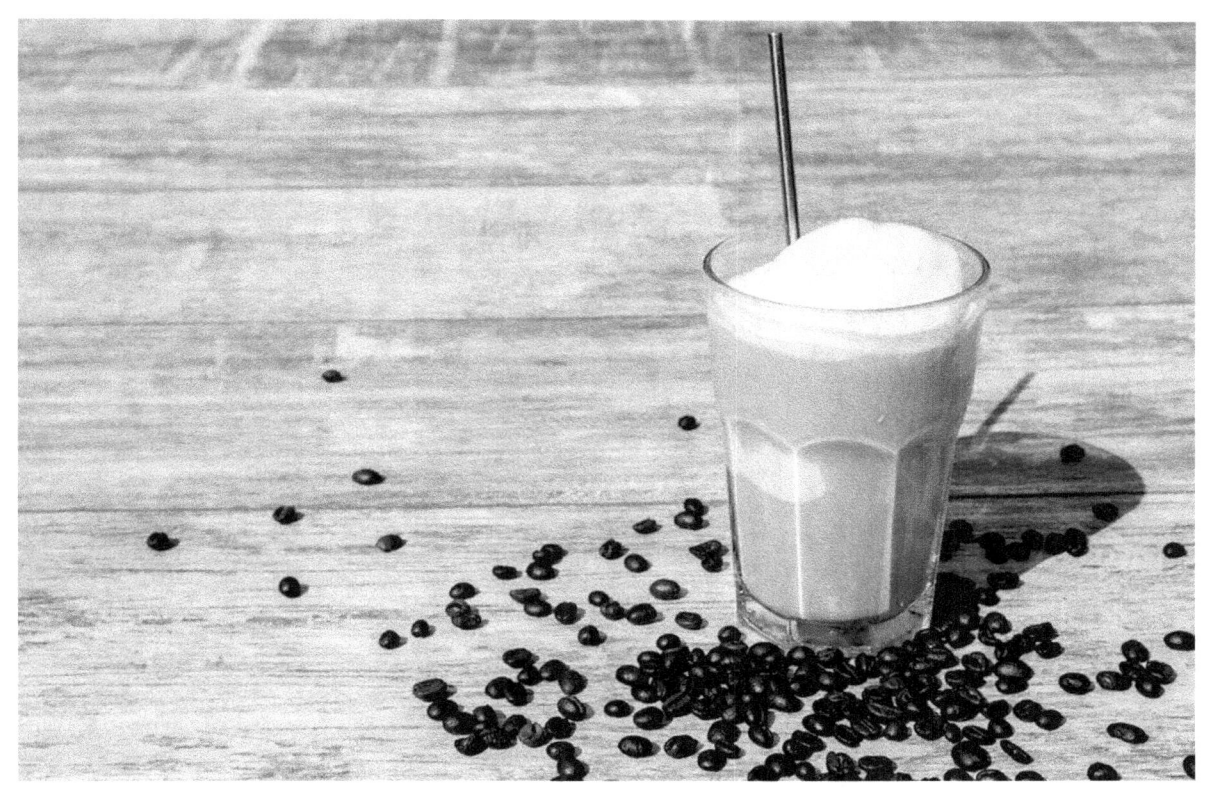

(**Freezer:** none / **Microwave:** none)

10. Mexican breakfast hash

(**Serves:** 2 / **Prep time:** 5 minutes / **Cooking time**: 20 minutes)

Nutritional Information (Per Serving)
Carbohydrates: 13.4 g
Fat: 34.9 g
Protein: 22.8 g
Calories: 25
Fiber: 6 g
Sodium: 89 mg

Ingredients
- Cilantro (fresh, garnish)
- Ghee (1 tablespoon)
- Avocados (1/2 cup, diced)
- Onion (1/2, chopped)
- Pepper (to taste)
- Green pepper (1/2, sliced)
- Eggs (2)
- Zucchini (1 cup, chopped)
- Mexican chorizo (6 ounces, remove the casing)
- Tomatoes (1/2 cup, chopped)
- Spinach (2 cups, chopped)

Instructions
1. Take a pan and smear it with ghee.
2. Toss in the onion and cook it on high before adding in the onion.
3. Allow the batter to cook for about three minutes before adding in the zucchini and tomatoes. Cook for another four minutes making sure to stir it so that it does not burn.

4. Now add the chorizo in and combine everything together.
5. After cooking for five minutes, the spinach will need to be added and cooked for three more minutes.
6. With a spatula, you will create two wells and crack your eggs into these wells.
7. Season to taste before moving the pan to the broiler. The hash will cook until the egg whites begin to set, and the yolks remain runny.
8. Top with avocado and cilantro before serving.

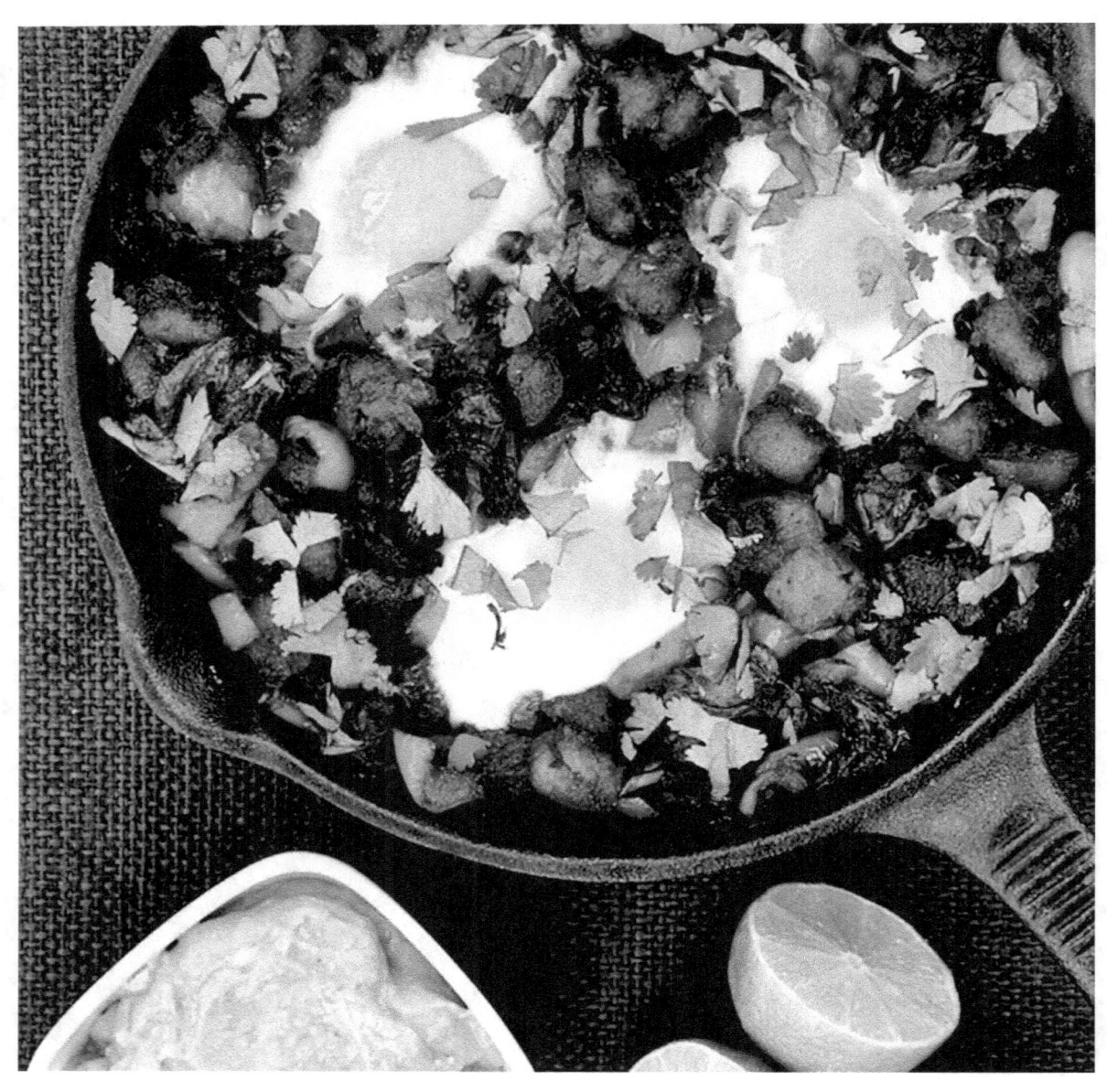

(**Freezer:** 1 month / **Microwave:** 1 ½ minutes)

11. Beef and pumpkin breakfast casserole

(**Serves:** 4 / **Prep time:** 20 minutes / **Cooking time:** 30 minutes)

Nutritional Information (Per Serving)
Calories: 386.6
Fat: 24.8 g
Protein: 23 g
Carbohydrates: 18.1 g
Fiber: 3.2 g
Sodium: 461 mg

Ingredients
- Pepper (to taste)
- Ground beef (17.6 ounces)
- Ghee (1.6 ounces)
- Onion (white, 1)
- Heavy whipping cream (.5 cup)
- Garlic (3 cloves)
- Eggs (6)
- Pumpkin (diced, 8.2 ounces)
- Cheddar cheese (shredded, 8 ounces)
- Mustard or Dijon mustard (1 tablespoon)

Instructions
1. Turn on your oven to 350 F.
2. Cook the beef in a pan that has been greased with ghee. Make sure to break any large pieces apart.
3. Cook until completely browned.
4. Place meat in a bowl and set aside.

5. Put the onion and the garlic the garlic should be cooked until it is browned. This will be about ten minutes of your time.
6. Cut up the pumpkin and put in the pan and cook until it has become fork tender.
7. Once done, set in the bowl with the ground beef and add in mustard of your choosing.
8. Mix in cheese until well combined.
9. Crack and mix eggs with cream and season to taste.
10. Place in a bowl.
11. Coat in egg mixture, so every inch of the beef and pumpkin is covered.
12. Use what cheese you have left over to cover the top of the egg mix.
13. Cook for twenty-five minutes.
14. Serve with sriracha sauce.

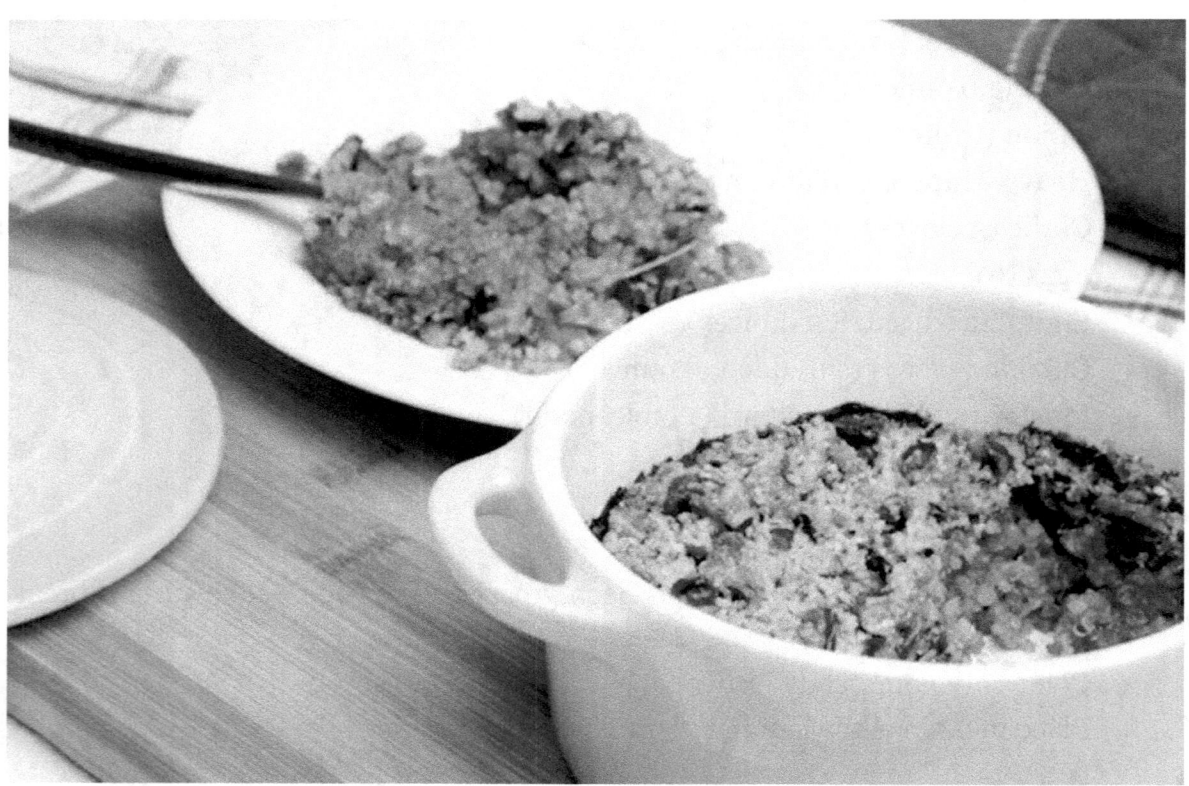

(**Freezer:** 8 months / **Microwave:** 3 ½ minutes)

12. Low carb lemon poppy seed muffins

(**Serves:** 8 / **Prep time:** 15 minutes / **Cooking time**: 15 minutes)

Nutritional Information (Per Serving)
Calories: 116
Fat: 4.8 g
Protein: 3.6 g
Carbohydrates: 10 g
Fiber: 0.8 g
Sodium: 240 mg

Ingredients
1. Heavy whipping cream (2 tablespoons)
2. Low-calorie natural sweetener (1/3 cup)
3. Vanilla extract (1/2 teaspoon)
4. Almond flour (1/4 cup)
5. Sour cream (2 tablespoons)
6. Coconut flour (1/4 cup)
7. Butter (3 tablespoons)
8. Poppy seeds (1 tablespoon)
9. Eggs (3)
10. Lemon (1, zested)
11. Xanthan gum (1/4 teaspoon)
12. Baking powder (1/2 teaspoon)
13. Salt (1/2 teaspoon)

Instructions
1. Preheat oven to 350 F. Take your muffin tin and spray with grease or place muffin liners inside of it.
2. Combine the flours, poppy seeds, sweetener, lemon zest, salt, xanthan gum, and baking powder in a bowl together.

3. Using your electric mixer, beat the eggs until they are fluffy. This is going to take around two minutes. After you have done that, you will beat the butter, vanilla extract, and sour cream into the mix. Then you are going to stir the cream in slowly until the batter is thick but smooth.
4. Pour into your muffin tin and try to make sure you are making the muffins even.
5. Bake for fifteen to twenty minutes or until the tops of the muffins are golden.

Soup and stew

1. Cauliflower soup with crumbled pancetta

(**Serves:** 4 / **Prep time:** 5 minutes / **Cooking time:** 15 minutes)

Nutritional Information (Per Serving)
Calories: 1052
Carbs: 22 g
Protein: 29 g
Fat: 94 g
Fiber: 4.2 g
Sodium: 853 mg

Ingredients
1. Pecan nuts (3 ½ ounces)
2. Chicken stock (3 ¾ cups)
3. Paprika (1 teaspoon)
4. Cauliflower (1 pound)
5. Butter (1 tablespoon, to be used for frying)
6. Cream cheese (7 ¾ ounces)
7. Pancetta (7 ¾ ounces, you can also use bacon)
8. Dijon mustard (1 tablespoon)
9. pepper (to taste)
10. Butter (4 ounces)

Instructions
1. Cut cauliflower into florets. The smaller you make them, the less time it will take for the soup to cook.
2. Save a handful and sauté with the pancetta in the frying butter.
3. Add in nuts and paprika.

4. Set aside, save the fat.
5. Put the rest of the cauliflower into the stock and allow to boil until soft.
6. Combine cream cheese, butter, and mustard in the pot.
7. Use a blender to mix to the consistency that you desire.
8. Season to taste.
9. Serve with pancetta and cauliflower crumbled on top.

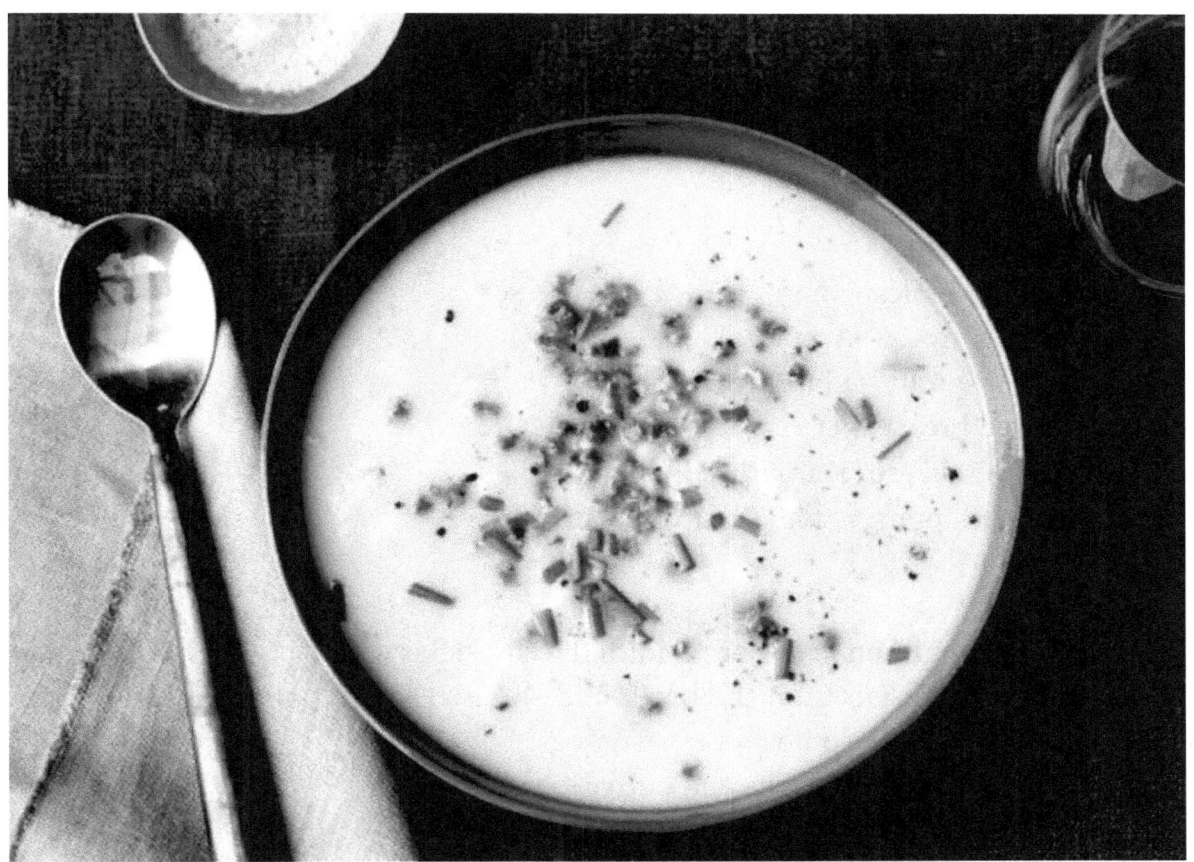

(**Freezer:** 5 months / **Microwave:** 3 ½ minutes)

2. Chicken soup

(**Serves:** 2 / **Prep time:** 5 minutes / **Cooking time:** 25 minutes)

Nutritional Information (Per Serving)
Calories: 1009
Carbs: 9 g
Protein: 119 g
Fat: 73 g
Fiber: 1.2 g
Sodium: 68 mg

Ingredients
1. Butter (6 tablespoons)
2. Chicken broth (32 ounces)
3. Brussel sprouts (1 bag, frozen)
4. Chicken breasts (3)
5. Cheddar cheese (1 cup, shredded)
6. Heavy whipping cream (1 cup)

Instructions
1. Boil your chicken in the broth until the chicken is done.
2. Take the chicken from the broth and shred it before putting it back in the pot. Season with some fajita seasonings.
3. Drop the Brussel sprouts and butter to your pan.
4. Allow simmering for about ten minutes.
5. Mix the whipping cream and cheese into the pot now.
6. Simmer another five minutes.

(**Freezer:** 4 months / **Microwave:** 3 minutes)

3. Eggplant and lamb soup

(Serves: 6 / **Prep time:** 10 minutes / **Cooking time:** 3 hours)

Nutritional Information (Per Serving)
Calories: 292
Protein: 18.2g
Fat: 16.2g
Carbs: 20.8g
Fiber: 8.4 g
Sodium: 871 mg

Ingredients
- Parsley (4 tablespoons, chopped)
- Eggplant (2)
- Cinnamon stick (1)
- Coconut oil (1 tablespoon)
- Turmeric (1/4 teaspoons)
- Lamb shanks (2 lb.)
- Garlic powder (1/2 teaspoons)
- Chicken broth (4 cups)
- Cumin (1/2 teaspoons)
- Water (2 cups)
- Sweet potato (1 pound)
- Onion (1, chopped)
- Garlic cloves (4)

Instructions
1. Turn the oven on to 400 F.
2. Poke holes in the eggplant that you have placed on a cookie sheet and cook for about sixty minutes.

3. Remove from oven and allow to cool.
4. Take the coconut oil and melt on medium.
5. Sear the lamb shanks in the oil.
6. Now add the water, onion, garlic, and broth.
7. Boil before reducing the temperature and simmering for an hour and a half.
8. Remove and let cool.
9. Toss potatoes and seasonings into the pot and stir as you bring it back to a boil.
10. Lower the heat again and allow to simmer for twenty-five minutes or until the potatoes have become soft.
11. Cut the lamb off the bones and into small pieces.
12. Peel the eggplant and remove skin.
13. Take the pan off the heat and get rid of the cinnamon stick.
14. Place the soup in a blender and blend until smooth.
15. Add in eggplant and mix again.
16. Put lamb in the soup and enjoy.

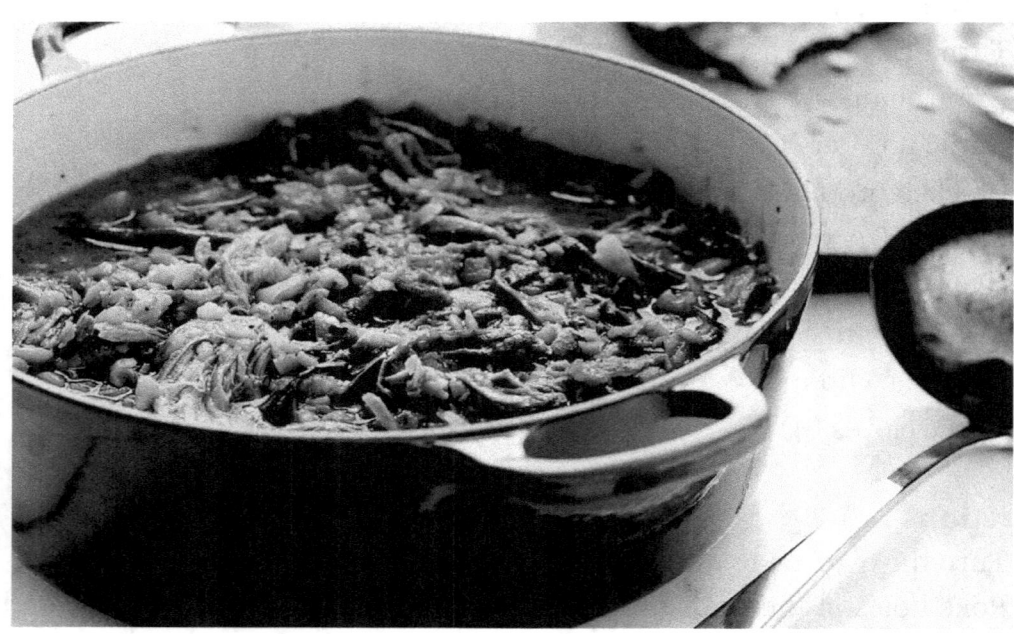

(**Freezer:** 2 months / **Microwave:** 2 ½ minutes)

4. Beef and winter vegetable soup

(Serves: 6 / **Prep time:** 15 minutes / **Cooking time:** 1 hour)

Health information (Per Serving)
Calories: 627
Carbs: 49 g
Protein: 40 g
Fat: 31 g
Fiber: 10.7 g
Sodium: 1000 mg

Ingredients
- Beef chuck roast (2 lbs., boneless)
- Cooking fat (spoonful)
- Onion (1/2 cup, chopped)
- Parsley (1 tablespoon, minced)
- Rutabaga (1, cubed)
- Thyme (1/2 teaspoons, dried)
- Sweet potatoes (2, cubed)
- Beef stock (6 c)
- Carrots (2, chunked)
- Garlic cloves (2, minced)
- Parsnip (2, chunked)
- Cauliflower (2 cups, riced)

Instructions
1. Melt the fat in a saucepan.
2. Brown the beef and set aside.
3. Toss in garlic and onion and cook for five minutes.
4. Add ½ of the stock in order to deglaze the pan.

5. Drop in all the vegetables and cook for about minute minutes
6. Re-add the beef to the pan and cover.
7. Simmer for forty-five minutes.
8. Sprinkle with seasonings.
9. Enjoy.

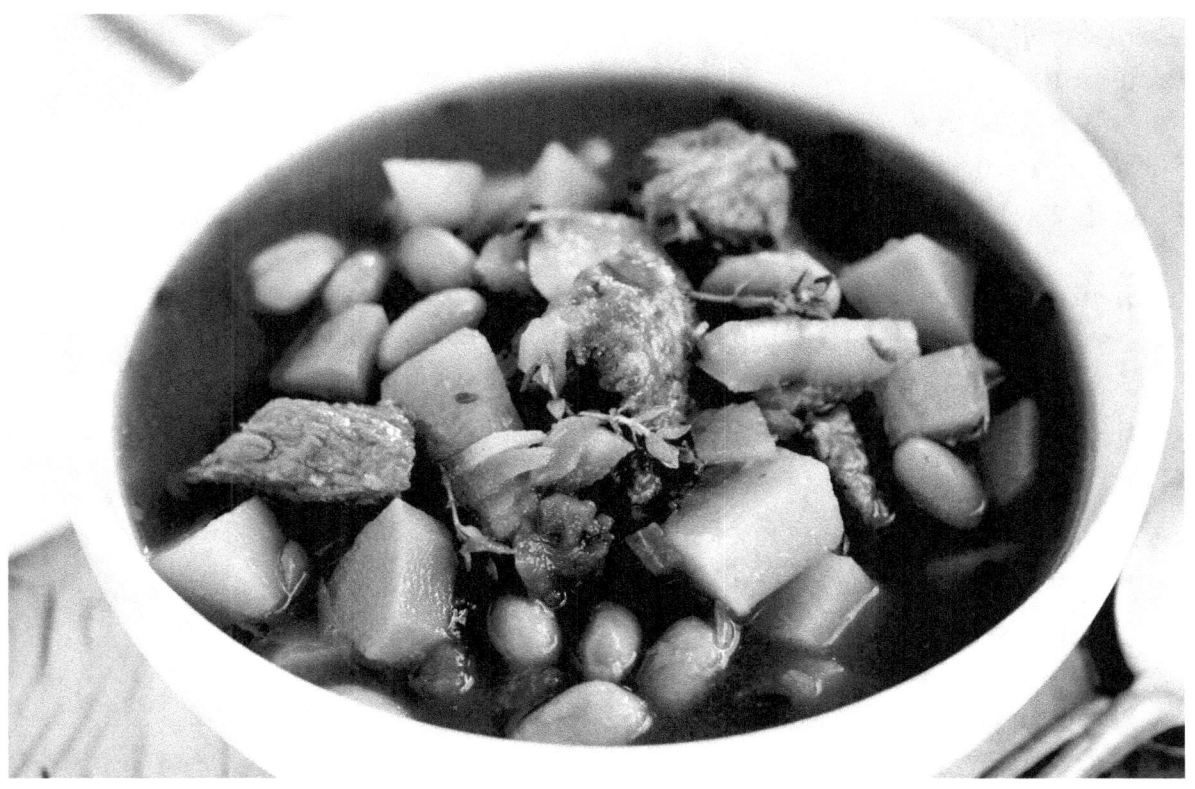

(**Freezer:** 2 months / **Microwave:** 1 ½ minutes)

5. Chicken and vegetable soup

(**Serves:** 8 / **Prep time:** 20 minutes / **Cooking time:** 25 minutes)

Nutritional Information (Per Serving)
Fat: 5 g
Calories: 98
Protein: 10 g
Carbohydrates: 11 g
Sodium: 319 mg
Fiber: 3.2 g

Shopping list
- Chicken (1.5 cups, shredded, cooked)
- Cauliflower (1 cup, chunked)
- Paleo approved cooking fat (2 tablespoons)
- Bell pepper (1, diced)
- Garlic cloves (3, minced)
- Leek (1, sliced)
- Chicken stock (8 cups)
- Onion (1, chopped)
- Parsley (1 handful, chopped)
- Zucchini (2, sliced)
- Bay leaves (2)
- Carrots (3, sliced)
- Thyme sprigs (4)
- Celery ribs (2, sliced)
- Tomatoes (1 cup, diced)

Instructions
1. Put a large stockpot on the stove over medium heat.

2. Cook onion, leek, garlic, chicken for five minutes.
3. Throw in the rest of the vegetables.
4. Add in chicken broth.
5. Cook until boiling.
6. Lower the temperature and simmer for twenty minutes.
7. Season to taste.

(**Freezer:** 2 months / **Microwave:** 2 minutes)

6. Easy spicy crockpot double beef stew

(**Serves:** 6 / **Prep time:** 5 minutes / **Cooking time:** 6 hours)

Nutritional Information (Per Serving)
Calories: 222
Fat: 7g
Protein: 27g
Carbohydrates: 11g
Fiber: 2 g
Sodium: 123 mg

Ingredients
- Worcestershire sauce (1 tablespoon)
- Beef stew meat (1.5 pounds)
- Hot sauce (2 teaspoons)
- Chili tomatoes (2 14.5 ounces)
- Chili mix (1 tablespoon)
- Beef broth (1 cup)

Instructions
1. Turn your crockpot on high.
2. Mix all of your ingredients together in your crockpot.
3. Cook for six hours.
4. Break up the meat after six hours.

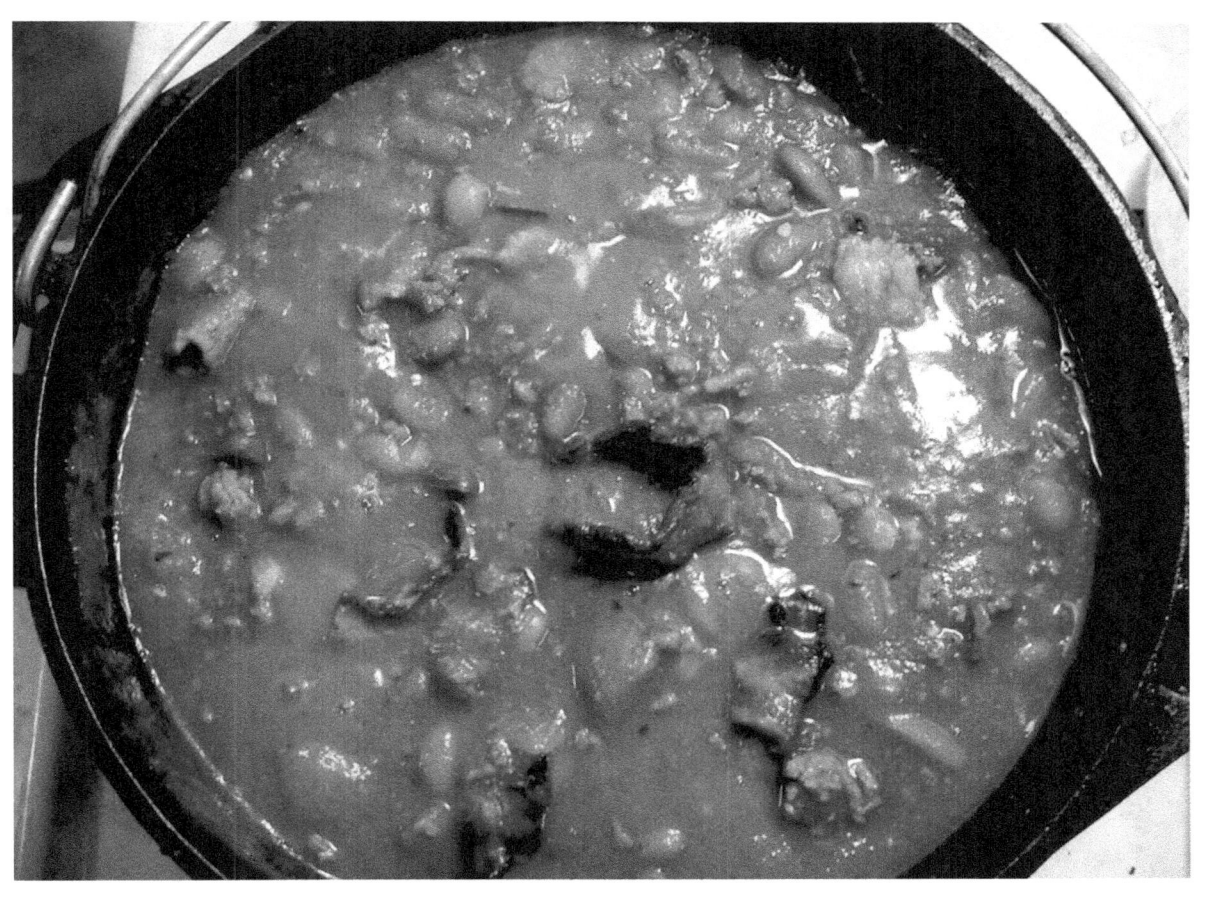

(**Freezer:** 3 months / **Microwave:** 2 minutes)

7. Chili soup

(**Serves:** 8 / **Prep time:** 5 minutes / **Cooking time:** 6 hours)

Nutritional Information (Per Serving)
Protein: 41 g
Carbohydrates: 7 g
Calories: 396
Fat: 21 g
Fiber: 9.4 g
Sodium: 830 mg

Ingredients
- Tomato paste (3 tablespoons)
- Butter (2 tablespoons)
- Coconut milk (unsweet, 0.25 cups)
- Onion (1)
- Beef stock (8 ounces)
- Pepper (1)
- Lemon juice (3 tablespoons)
- Ground pepper (16 ounces)
- Coconut flour (1 tablespoon)
- Bacon (8 slices, optional)
- Garlic (minced, 1 tablespoon)
- Thyme (1 tablespoon)
- Pepper (1 teaspoon)
- (1 teaspoon)
-

Instructions
1. Put butter in the center of the crockpot to melt.
2. Place onions and peppers in the bottom of the crockpot.

3. Place in ground beef.
4. Place bacon strips if you are using them.
5. Add in all seasonings.
6. Add in liquids.
7. Cover with tomato paste.
8. To cook, cover the top and cook for about six hours.
9. Stir to mix everything together.
10. Top with cheese.

(**Freezer:** 6 months / **Microwave:** 3 minutes)

8. Grandma's spaghetti soup

(**Serves:** 8 / **Prep time:** 10 minutes / **Cooking time:** 1 hour)

Nutritional Information (Per Serving)
Calories: 472
Fat: 21. 4 g
Protein: 20.8 g
Carbohydrates: 48.8 g
Sodium: 1446 mg
Fiber: 2.5 g

Ingredients
- Garlic powder (1/4 tsp)
- Italian sausage (1 lb.)
- Pepper (1/4 tsp)
- Ground beef (1 lb.)
- (1/2 tsp)
- Tomatoes (30 oz., diced)
- Oregano (1/2 tsp, dried)
- Beef broth (4 c)
- Basil (1/2 tsp, dried)
- Zucchini (1 lb., diced)
- Italian seasoning (1 tsp)
- Bell pepper (1, green, diced)
- Onion (1/2, chopped)
- Celery (1 c, sliced)

Instructions
1. Brown the meat.
2. Drain the meat.

3. Add the remaining ingredients in the pot.
4. Cook for an hour, until vegetables are tender.

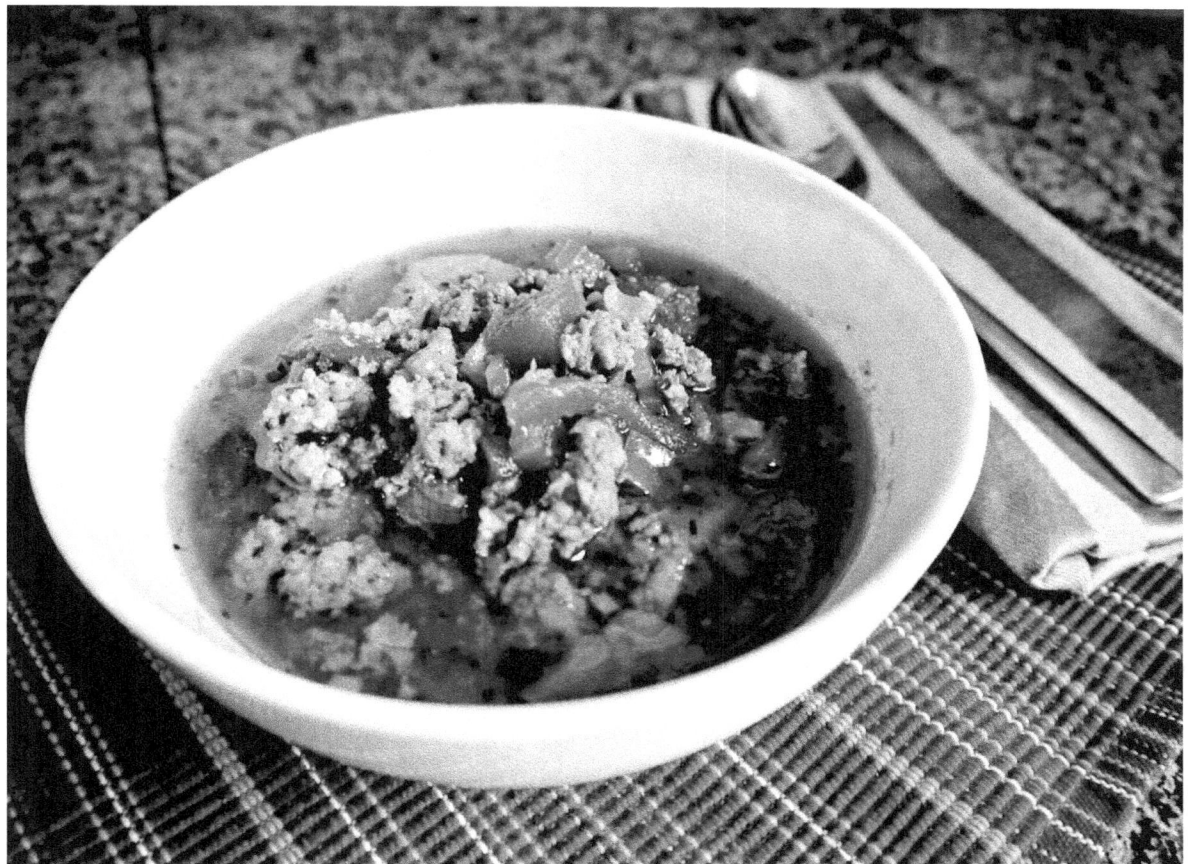

(**Freezer:** 3 months / **Microwave:** 2 minutes)

9. Meatball noodle soup

(**Serves:** 6 / **Prep time:** 10 minutes / **Cooking time:** 50 minutes)

Nutritional Information (Per Serving)
Fat: 14 g
Protein: 26 g
Calories: 278
Carbohydrates: 11 g
Fiber: 8.4 g
Sodium: 215 mg

Ingredients

Meatballs
- Egg yolks (2)
- Broth (2 c)
- Black pepper (1/2 tsp)
- Ground beef (1 lb.)
- (2 tsp)
- Onion (1/2 c, chopped)
- Parsley (1 tbsp, dried)
- Ghee (2 tbsp)

Soup
- Spaghetti squash (1, scraped clean)
- Broth (6 c)
- Carrot (1, chopped, peeled)
- Mushrooms (4, sliced)
- Onion (1/2 c, chopped)

Instructions
1. Sauté the ½ c onion in your ghee.
2. Mix in the ground beef, egg, pepper, and parsley.
3. Simmer 2 c of broth.
4. Roll your meat into meatballs and simmer in the broth until cooked.
5. Dump in 6 c broth, onions, carrots, and mushrooms.
6. Simmer until vegetables are soft.
7. Serve inside of a bowl with spaghetti squash

(**Freezer:** 8 months / **Microwave:** 3 minutes)

10. Pumpkin and chorizo soup

(**Serves:** 4 / **Prep time:** 10 minutes / **Cooking time:** 25 minutes)

Nutritional Information (Per Serving)
Calorie: 433
Fat: 35.1 g
Carbohydrates: 26 g
Protein 8.2 g
Sodium: 160.2 mg
Fiber: 6.3 g

Ingredients
- Cilantro (chopped)
- Olive oil (1 tbsp)
- pepper (to taste)
- Onion (1, diced)
- Chorizo sausage (1/2 lb., ground)
- Garlic cloves (4, minced)
- Chicken broth (3 c)
- Marjoram (1 tsp, dried)
- Pumpkin puree (30 oz.)
- Oregano (1 tsp, dried)
- Cumin (1/2 tsp)

Instructions
1. Put the olive oil in a skillet.
2. Sauté the onions.
3. Mix in the garlic and other spices. Cook for thirty seconds.
4. Dump in broth and puree. Simmer for twenty minutes covered.
5. Sauté the chorizo.

6. Blend soup together in the blender.
7. Place back in skillet and mix in sausage.
8. Enjoy with a little bit of cilantro.

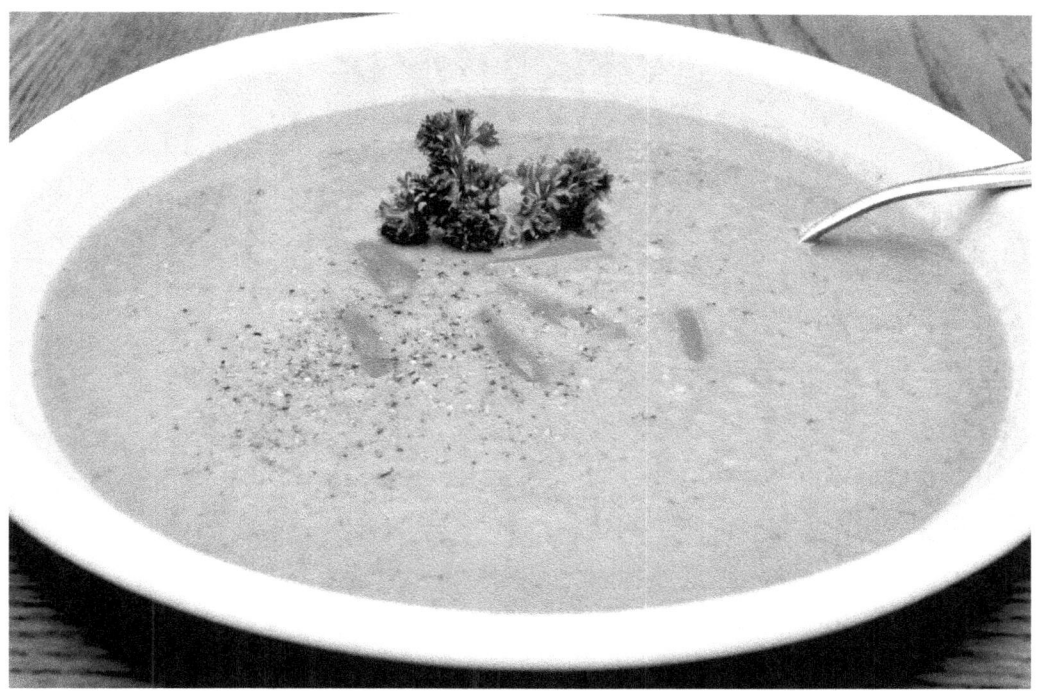

(**Freezer:** 3 months / **Microwave:** 2 minutes)

11. Orange ginger squash soup

(Serves: 4 / **Prep time:** 10 minutes / **Cooking time:** 1 hour)

Nutritional Information (Per Serving)
Calories: 180
Fat: 7 g
Carbohydrates: 28 g
Protein: 3 g
Sodium: 172 mg
Fiber: 6.9 g

Ingredients
- Almonds (sliced, optional)
- Pomegranate seeds (optional)
- Acorn squash (1)
- Cayenne pepper (a pinch)
- Olive oil (1/2 tsp)
- Coconut aminos (1 tbsp)
- pepper (to taste)
- Ginger (3/4 tsp, ground)
- Chicken stock (2 c)
- Orange zest (1 tsp)
- Coconut milk (1/4 c)
- Orange juice (1/4 c, fresh)

Instructions
1. Heat your oven to 400F.
2. Slice the squash in half and remove seeds and pulp.
3. Cover with olive oil and sprinkle with pepper.

4. Put on a pan and roast until tender. This could take about an hour.
5. As soon as the squash cools down, remove it from the flesh and put it in a saucepan or blender.
6. Toss in the remaining ingredients.
7. Blend until it is entirely smooth.
8. Cook until hot.
9. Serve with almonds or pomegranate seeds.

(**Freezer:** 6 months / **Microwave:** 2 ½ minutes)

12. Chicken bacon crock pot chowder

(**Serves:** 8 / **Prep time:** 20 minutes / **Cooking time:** 8 hours)

Nutritional Information (Per Serving)
Carbohydrates: 6.4 g
Calories: 355
Protein: 21 g
Fat: 28 g
Fiber: 62 g
Sodium: 489 mg

Ingredients

- Thyme (1 tsp, dried)
- Garlic cloves (4, minced)
- Garlic powder (1 tsp)
- Shallot (1, chopped)
- Black pepper (1 tsp)
- Leek (1, sliced)
- (1 tsp)
- Celery (2, diced)
- Bacon (1 lb., cooked and crumbled)
- Cremini mushrooms (6 oz., sliced)
- Heavy cream (1 c)
- Onion (1, sliced)
- Cream cheese (8 oz.)
- Butter (4 tbsp, divided)
- Chicken breasts (1 lb.)
- Chicken stock (2 c, divided)

Instructions
1. Turn your slow cooker on to low
2. Throw in the vegetables, stock, and pepper. Cook for an hour.
3. Sear the chicken in a skillet with the last of the butter this will be about five minutes.
4. Remove from pan and deglaze with last of the chicken stock.
5. Dump the chicken stock into the crockpot.
6. Add in heavy cream, cream cheese, thyme, garlic powder. Stir
7. After the chicken is no longer hot; cube and throw in the slow cooker.
8. Stir until all ingredients are mixed together.
9. Cover and cook for 6 hours.

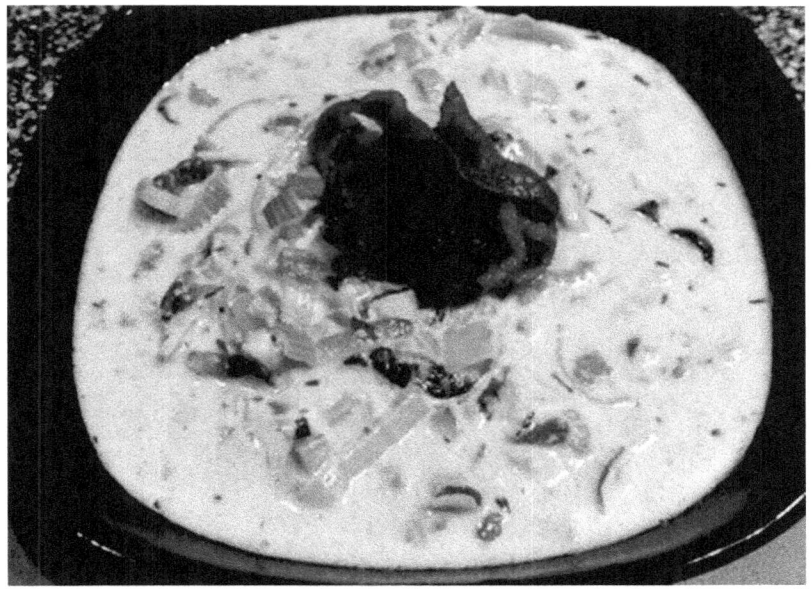

(**Freezer:** 3 months / **Microwave:** 3 minutes)

13. Thai coconut turkey soup

(**Serves:** 4 / **Prep time:** 10 minutes / **Cooking time:** 15 minutes)

Nutritional Information (Per Serving)
Calories: 172
Carbohydrates: 11 g
Protein: 17 g
Fat: 6 g
Fiber: 2 g
Sodium: 456 mg

Ingredients
- Sriracha (optional)
- Oil (a splash)
- (to taste)
- Onion (1, sliced) sprouts (2 handfuls)
- Shiitake mushrooms (handful, chopped)
- Bell pepper (1, any color)
- Garlic cloves (3, minced)
- Soy sauce (1 tbsp)
- Ginger (1, julienned)
- Thai curry paste (1 ½ tbsp., green)
- Cherry tomatoes (handful)
- Coconut milk (1/2 c)
- Turkey stock (4 c)
- Turkey (1 c, cooked)

Instructions
1. Put the oil in a pan and heat.
2. Drop in the onion and allow to cook until it becomes soft.

3. Now add in the mushrooms and cook for five minutes.
4. Lastly toss in the garlic, ginger, and tomatoes.
5. Now add in your meat, stock, milk and soy sauce along with the curry paste.
6. Allow boiling before reducing and simmering for two minutes.
7. Take off the heat and add the bell pepper and sprouts.
8. Season if you need to.
9. Put in a bowl and add in cilantro and sriracha if you want.

(**Freezer:** 1 month / **Microwave:** 1 ½ minutes)

14. Creamy white chili

(**Serves:** 8 / **Prep time:** 15 minutes / **Cooking time:** 40 minutes)

Nutritional Information (Per Serving)
Calories: 334
Fat: 7.9 g
Protein: 21.3 g
Carbohydrates: 29.7 g
Fiber: 6.4 g
Sodium: 888 mg

Ingredients
1. Heavy whipping cream (1/2 cup)
2. Olive oil (1 tablespoon)
3. Sour cream (1 cup)
4. Chicken breast (1 pound)
5. Cayenne pepper (1/4 teaspoon)
6. Onion (1, chopped)
7. Black pepper (1/2 teaspoon)
8. Garlic clove (2, chopped)
9. Oregano (1 teaspoon, dried)
10. Northern beans (2 15.5 ounce cans)
11. Cumin (1 teaspoon)
12. Chicken broth (14.5 ounces)
13. Salt (1 teaspoon)
14. Green chilies (2 4 ounce cans)

Instruction
1. Take a large saucepan and heat olive oil on a medium heat. Take your chicken and cook it while stirring in onion and garlic. Make sure that the

chicken is no longer pink before you move on to the next step. This step is going to take around fifteen minutes.
2. Mix your beans, chicken broth, spices, and chilies into the chicken. You should allow it to boil before you reduce the heat and simmer it until the flavors are blended.
3. Take the chili off the heat and stir in the sour cream along with the whipping cream until it is incorporated.

Vegetarian Mains

1. ## Chia Seed Crackers and roasted red pepper and goat cheese dip

(**Serves:** 36 crackers / **Prep time:** 15 minutes / **Cooking time:** 40 minutes)

Nutritional Information (Per Serving)
Calories: 28.17
Fat: 2.15g
Carbohydrates: 0.28g
Protein: 0.88g
Fiber: 1 g
Sodium: 390 mg

Ingredients
- Pepper (1/4 teaspoon)
- Chia seeds (1/2 cup, ground)
- (1/4 teaspoon)
- Cheddar cheese (3 ounces, shredded)
- Paprika (1/4 teaspoon)
- Ice water (1 ¼ cup)
- Oregano (1/4 teaspoon)
- Psyllium husk powder (2 tablespoons)
- Onion powder (1/4 teaspoon)
- Olive oil (2 tablespoons)
- Garlic powder (1/4 teaspoon)
- Xanthan gum (1/4 teaspoon)

Instructions
1. Turn your oven on to 375 F.

2. Place the chia seeds in a spice grinder and grind them down to a meal like texture.
3. Add the husk powder, the gum, garlic powder, oregano, onion powder, paprika, and pepper into a bowl and make sure that you mix it all so that all the spices are incorporated thoroughly, and you do not see any of the spices individually.
4. Add your olive oil to the dry mixture and create what will appear to be wet sand.
5. Now mix the ice water into the bowl. You will want to make sure that the seeds and the husk powder really absorbs the water so that dough is formed.
6. Grate your cheese and toss it into the bowl as well.
7. Knead your dough together. Your dough needs to be dry rather than sticky when you have finished kneading the dough.
8. Take the dough out of a bowl and place it on a piece of parchment paper so that it can settle for a few moments.
9. Spread the dough out after allowing it to sit so that it covers the entire piece of parchment paper. You can make it as thin as you want to.
10. Bake for thirty-five minutes
11. Once done, take them out of the oven and cut them while they are still hot so that they become individual crackers.
12. Throw your crackers back in the oven for another five minutes or until they are brown and crispy.

2. Roasted red pepper and goat cheese dip

(**Serves:** 6 / **Prep time:** 5 minutes / **Cooking time:** 10 minutes)

Nutritional Information (Per Serving)
Calories: 393.5
Fat: 32.9g
Carbohydrate: 14.5g
Protein: 13 g
Sodium: 224 mg
Fiber: 0.1 g

Ingredients
- Goat cheese (8 ounces)
- Red bell peppers (2)
- Black pepper (1 teaspoon)
- Garlic clove (1)
- Kosher (1 teaspoon)
- Olive oil (6 tablespoons)
- Rosemary (2 tablespoons, dried)
- Basil (2 tablespoons, dried)
- Oregano (4 tablespoons, dried)

Instructions
1. Slice your peppers in half and place them in a pan with the side that you. Cut up and drizzle about two tablespoons of oil over them before sprinkling with.
2. Place in the oven at 375 F and cook until the skin begins to blister. Once this happens, you will remove them from the oven and take the skins off once the peppers have cooled.
3. Now you will take the peppers, cheese, and garlic cloves and place them into the food processor. You are going to need to pulse these ingredients together until they create a smooth paste.

4. Now add in your olive oil, herbs, and season. Continue to pulse until it is well blended.
5. Put in a bowl and stir until it is homogenized.
6. Place in the fridge for about two hours before serving. It should be covered when placed in the refrigerator.

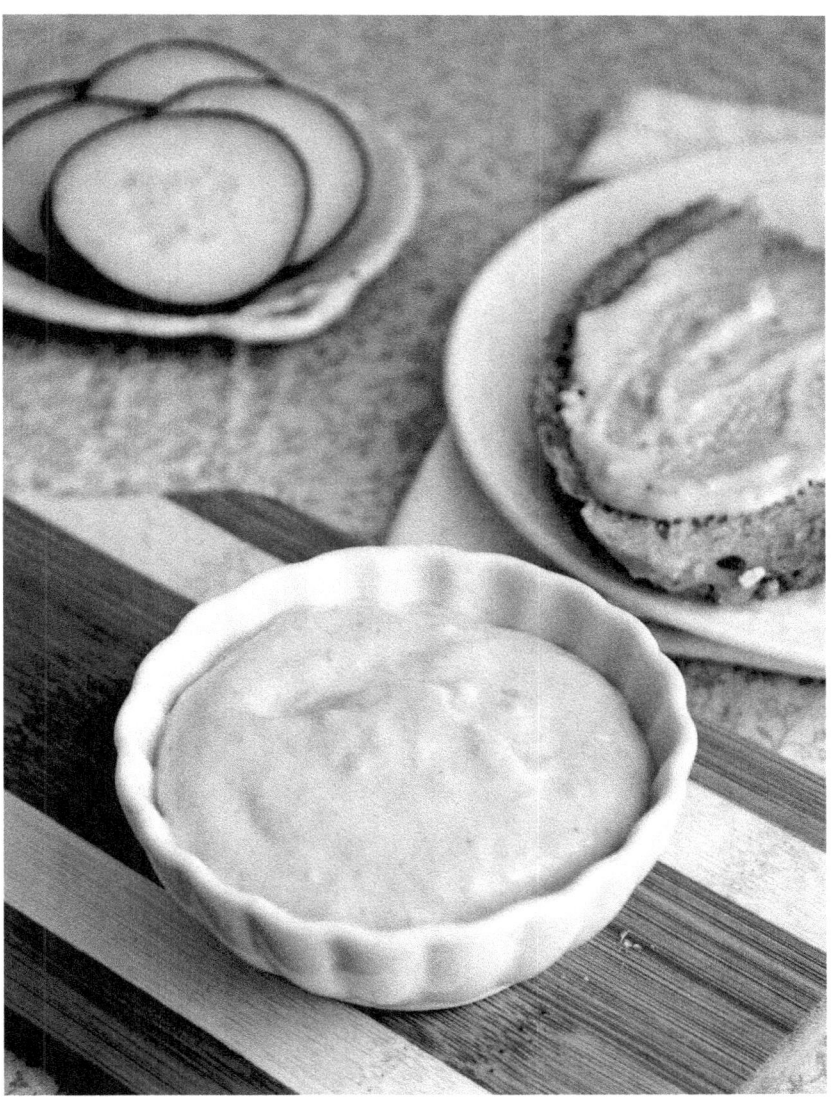

(**Freezer:** none / **Microwave:** none)

3. Multi-purpose mini loaves with carrots and thyme

(**Serves:** 4 / **Prep time:** 10 minutes / **Cooking time:** 45 minutes)

Nutritional Information (Per Serving)
Calories: 20
Fat: 33.7g
Protein: 12.7 g
Fiber: 2 g
Sodium: 231 mg
Carbohydrates: 17.3g

Ingredients
- Sea salt (to taste)
- Carrots (4)
- Thyme (2 tablespoons)
- Flaxseed (2.1 ounces, blitzed)
- Eggs (2)
- Pumpkin seeds (1.8 ounces)
- Olive oil (3 tablespoons)
- Sunflower seeds (1.4 ounces)

Instructions
1. Preheat your oven to 375 F before taking 4 mini baking pans and greasing them with some oil.
2. Blitz the carrots so that they start to look like rice.
3. Take a fork and whisk your eggs before adding in your carrots, flaxseed, sunflower seeds, pumpkin seeds, olive oil, and fresh thyme.
4. Using a spoon, put the mix into your loaf pans and cook for around forty-five minutes. Drizzle with some of the toasted sesame oil and a sprig of fresh thyme.

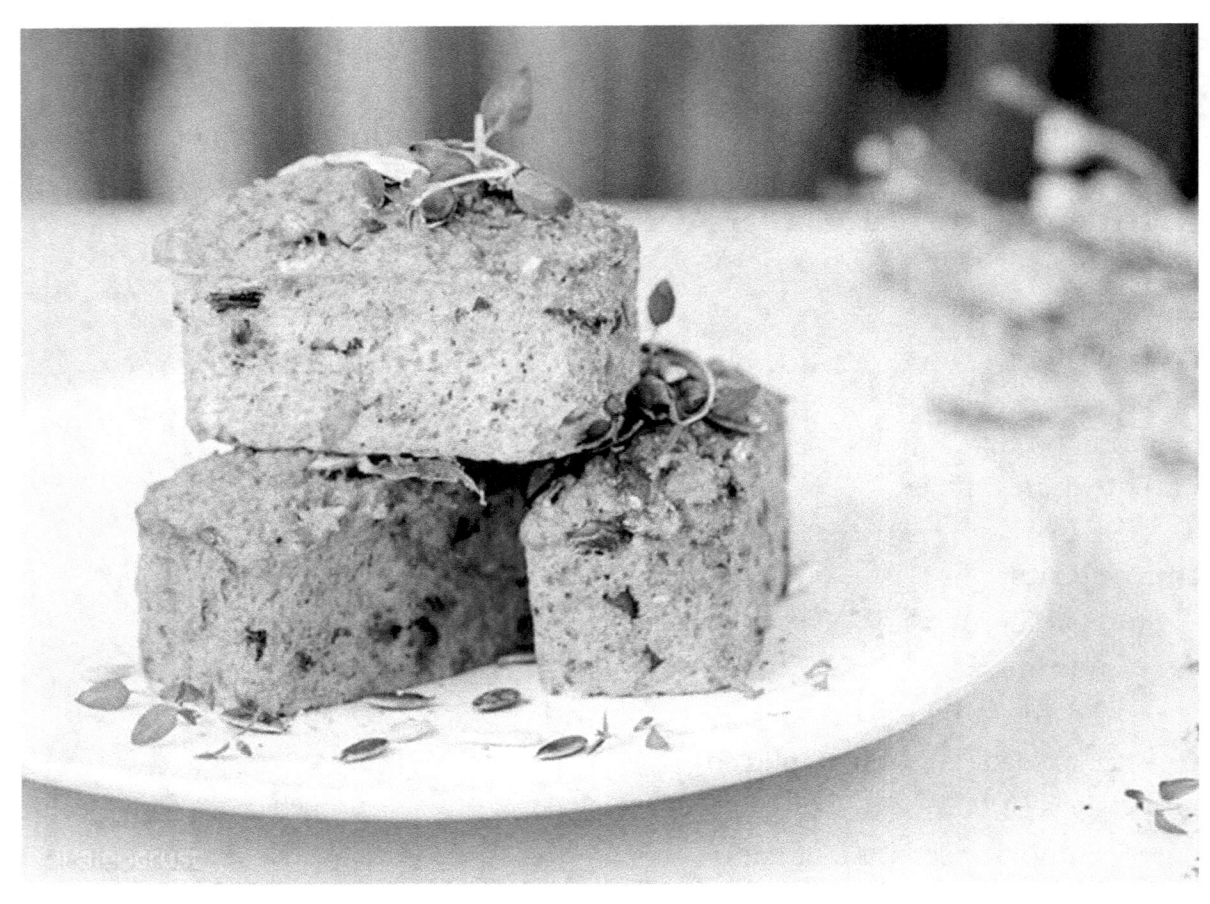

(**Freezer:** 6 months / **Microwave:** none)

4. Egg drop soup

(**Serves:** 4 / **Prep time:** 10 minutes / **Cooking time:** 10 minutes)

Nutritional Information (Per Serving)
Calories: 76
Fat: 4.1g
Protein: 4.9 g
Carbohydrates: 4.2 g
Sodium: 1143 mg
Fiber: 0.1 g

Ingredients
- Olive oil (6 tablespoons)
- Chicken stock (2 quarts)
- Black pepper (to taste)
- Turmeric (1 tablespoon, fresh, grated)
- Ginger (1 tablespoon, raw, grated)
- Cilantro (2 tablespoons, fresh, chopped)
- Garlic cloves (2, minced)
- Spring onions (2, sliced)
- Chile pepper (1, sliced)
- Eggs (4)
- Coconut aminos (2 tablespoons)
- Spinach (4 cups, chopped)
- Brown mushrooms (2 cups, sliced)

Instructions
1. Dump the chicken stock into a pot and heat it up, so it begins to simmer. While this is happening, slice your mushrooms and the spinach. Dump the

seasonings, herbs, and vegetables in the pot along with the coconut aminos. They should be allowed to simmer for about five minutes.
2. Take the eggs and whisk them in a bowl before pouring them into the soup.
3. Stir while the eggs cook and then take off of the heat. Chop your cilantro up and slice the onion. Add this to your pot.
4. Drizzle with olive oil after you have poured it into a bowl.

(**Freezer:** 1 month / **Microwave:** 2 minutes)

5. Low carb Greek briam

(**Serves:** 6 / **Prep time:** 30 minutes / **Cooking time:** 15 minutes)

Nutritional Information (Per Serving)
Calories: 76
Carbohydrates: 13.9g
Protein: 8.7g
Fat: 35.8 g
Fiber: 4.7 g
Sodium: 45 mg

Ingredients
- Olive oil (1/2 cup)
- Onion (1, sliced)
- Feta cheese (1 ½ cup, crumbled)
- Garlic cloves (2, minced)
- Black pepper (to taste)
- Ghee (1/4 cup)
- (1/4 teaspoon)
- Eggplant (1, diced)
- Oregano (1 tablespoon, chopped)
- Cauliflower (1/2, chopped)
- Parsley (1/4 cup, chopped)
- Broccoli (1/2, chopped)
- Zucchini (2, sliced)
- Green pepper (1, sliced)
- Vegetable stock (1/4 cup)
- Tomato (3, chopped)

Instructions
1. Crush your garlic and peel your onion. In a casserole dish, you are going to put down your ghee and cook the onion and garlic for five minutes.
2. As this is happening, dice up your eggplant, after the onion and garlic have browned, you will put the eggplant in with them and place a lid on it so that it can cook for three minutes.
3. Cut the florets of the cauliflower and broccoli
4. Toss into the dish and mix before recovering and cooking for three minutes.
5. Cut up your pepper, and tomato. Toss that into the dish as well. Now add the stock and cover once more. Cook for another five minutes.
6. While this cook, slice your zucchini before adding that in.
7. Next, the seasonings need to go in.
8. Put under a broiler that you have already preheated and allow the cheese to become lightly browned.
9. Garnish with the parsley after drizzling with olive oil.

(**Freezer:** 2 months / **Microwave:** 45 seconds)

6. Saffron cauliflower soup with sumac oil

(**Serves:** 8 cups / **Prep time**: 5 minutes / **Cooking time:** 1 hour 10 minutes)

Nutritional Information (Per Serving)
Protein: 2.6 g
Cholesterol: none
Calories: 70
Fat: 3.8 g
Fiber: 1 g
Sodium: 716 mg

Ingredients
- Saffron threads (20)
- Olive oil (2 tbsp)
- Water or vegetable broth (5 c)
- Onion (1, chopped)
- Pepper (1/4 tsp)
- Garlic cloves (2, chopped)
- (1/2 tsp)
- Cauliflower florets (2 lbs., fresh or frozen)

Instructions
1. Take your garlic and onion and sauté it in the olive oil on medium-high heat for around ten minutes.
2. Toss in the cauliflower and the pepper. Cook for another twelve minutes.
3. Add your liquid and allow to boil until the cauliflower is tender. This could take up to twenty-five minutes.
4. Take off the heat and stir in the saffron before covering the pot.
5. Saffron should be able to steep for around twenty minutes.
6. Dump into the blender and blend until it is a creamy mixture.
7. Serve with a little bit of sumac oil (if you want).

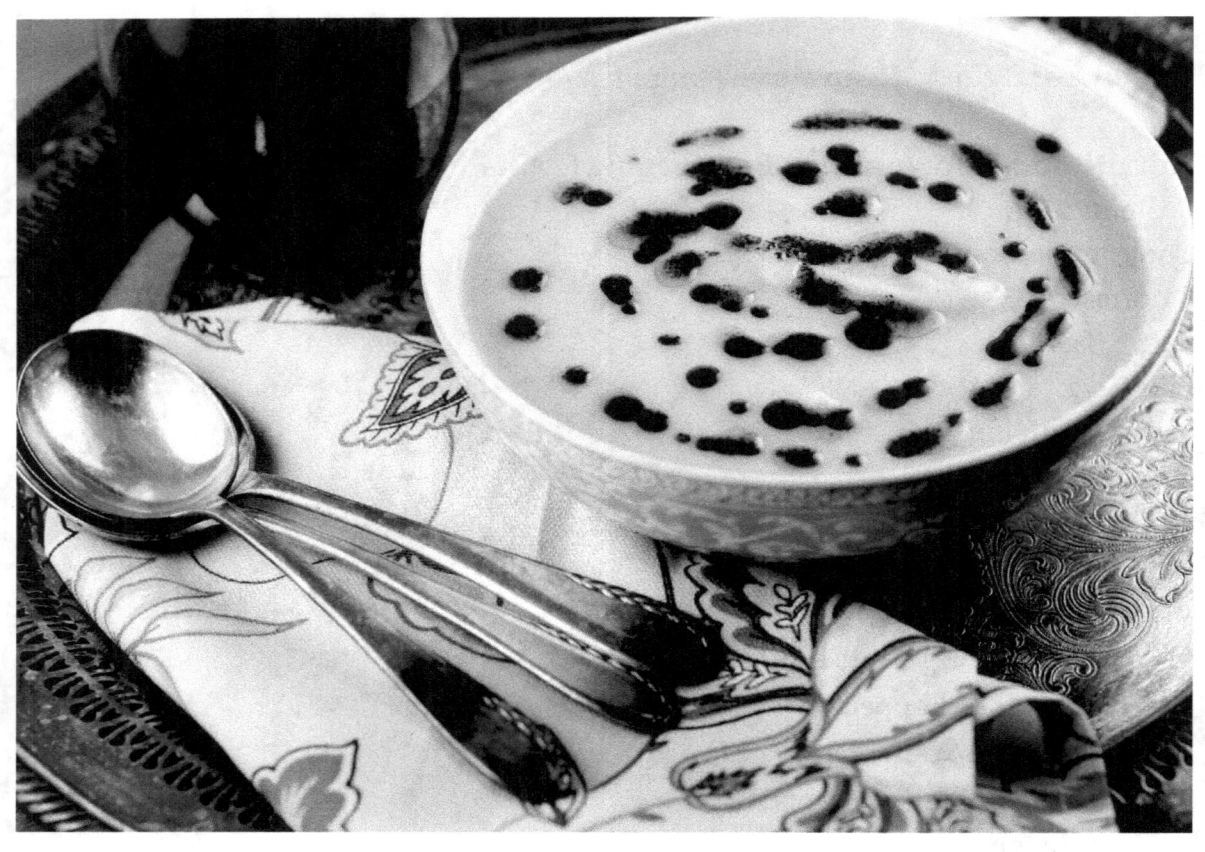

(**Freezer:** 6 months / **Microwave:** 45 seconds)

7. Roasted broccoli salad

(**Serves:** 2 / **Prep time:** 5 minutes / **Cooking time:** 25 minutes)

Nutritional Information (Per Serving)
Fat: 28 g
Protein: 4.50 g
Carbohydrates: 13 g
Calories: 299
Fiber: 4.2 g
Sodium: 128 mg

Ingredients
- Onion (1, halved, sliced)
- Broccoli (4 c, cut into small pieces)
- Oregano (1 tsp)
- Cherry tomatoes (2 c)
- Balsamic vinegar (1 tbsp)
- Coconut oil (1 tbsp)
- Onion (4, green, chopped)
- Garlic cloves (2, minced)

Instructions
1. Turn your oven on to 375 F.
2. Put the oil, garlic, onion, tomato, and broccoli in a bowl and coat.
3. Spread out on a cookie sheet and cook for twenty-five minutes.
4. Put back in a bowl and put the rest of the ingredients in.

(**Freezer:** 1 month / **Microwave:** 1 minute 15 seconds)

8. Apple, pear, and walnut salad

(**Serves:** 2 / **Prep time:** 5 minutes / **Cooking time:** none)

Nutritional Information (Per Serving)
Calories: 258
Fat: 20.7 g
Sodium: 475 mg
Carbohydrates: 15.2 g
Fiber: 3.2 g
Protein: 6.1 g

Ingredients
- Walnuts (1/2 c)
- Apples (2, diced, peeled)
- Cinnamon (1/2 tsp)
- Pears (2, diced, peeled)
- Raisins (1/3 c)
- Orange juice (1/3 c)

Instructions
1. Mix everything together
2. Put in the fridge for an hour
3. Enjoy!

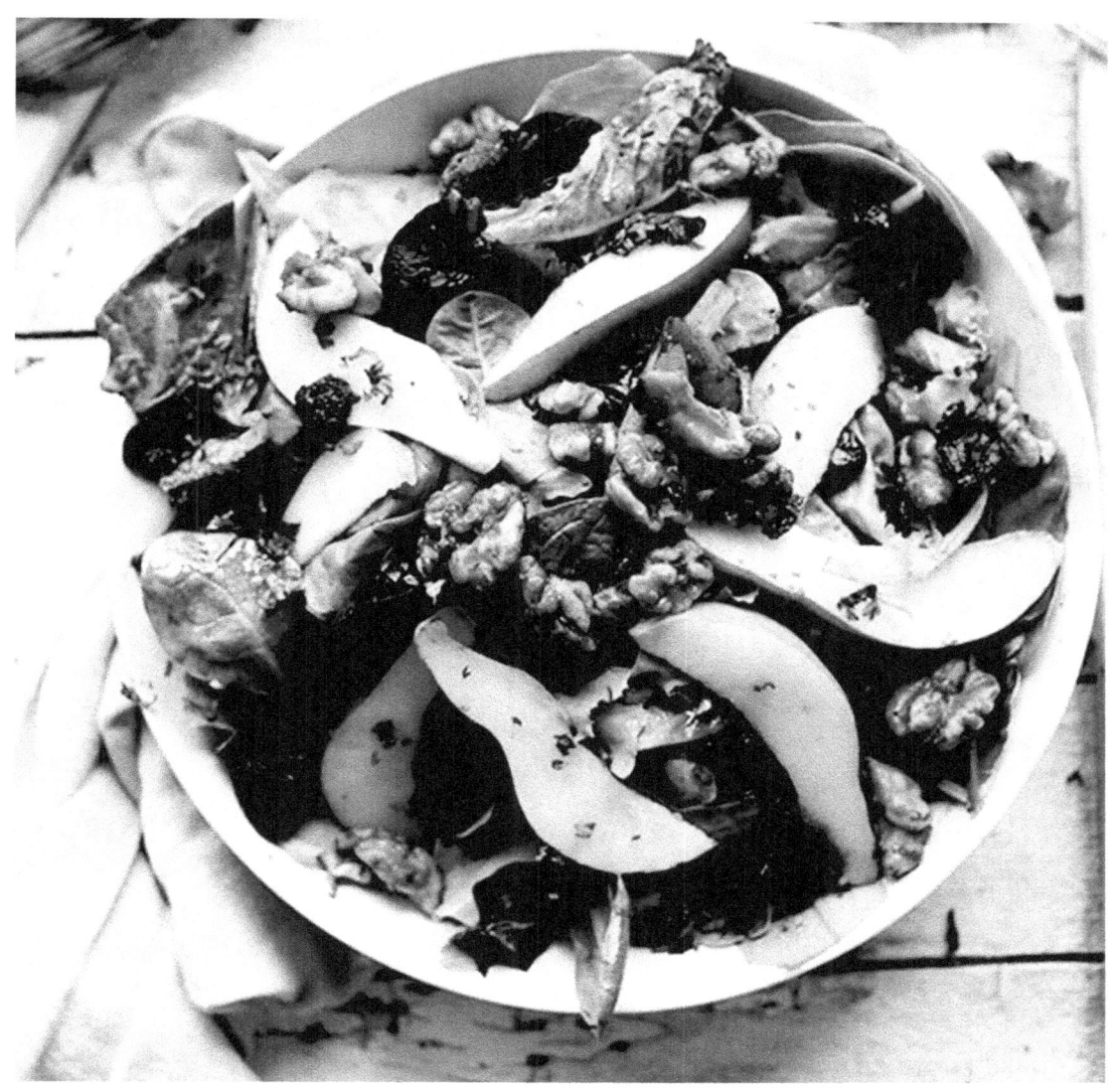

9. Pesto egg salad wrap

(**Serves:** 3 / **Prep time:** 10 minutes / **Cooking time:** 15 minutes)

Nutritional Information (Per Serving)
Calories: 160
Carbohydrate: 2 g
Fat: 3 g
Protein: 9 g
Sodium: 172 mg
Fiber: 0 g

Ingredients

Wraps
- Pesto (1/3 c)
- Eggs (3, hardboiled)
- Cucumber (1/4, diced)
- Collard leaves (3, large)

Pesto
- Sea salt (to taste)
- Basil (1 bunch)
- Lemon juice (1/2 c)
- Olive oil (1 c)
- Walnuts (1/2 c)

Instructions
1. Remove the stems from the collard leaves.
2. Heat about half an inch of water in a skillet over high heat.
3. Place your leaves in and cover so that they cook until they are wilted.

4. Allow drying while you mix the pesto, eggs, and cucumbers together.
5. Place in the leaf and roll as if it was a burrito.

Pesto
1. Put everything in the food processor and blend together.
2. Season to taste.

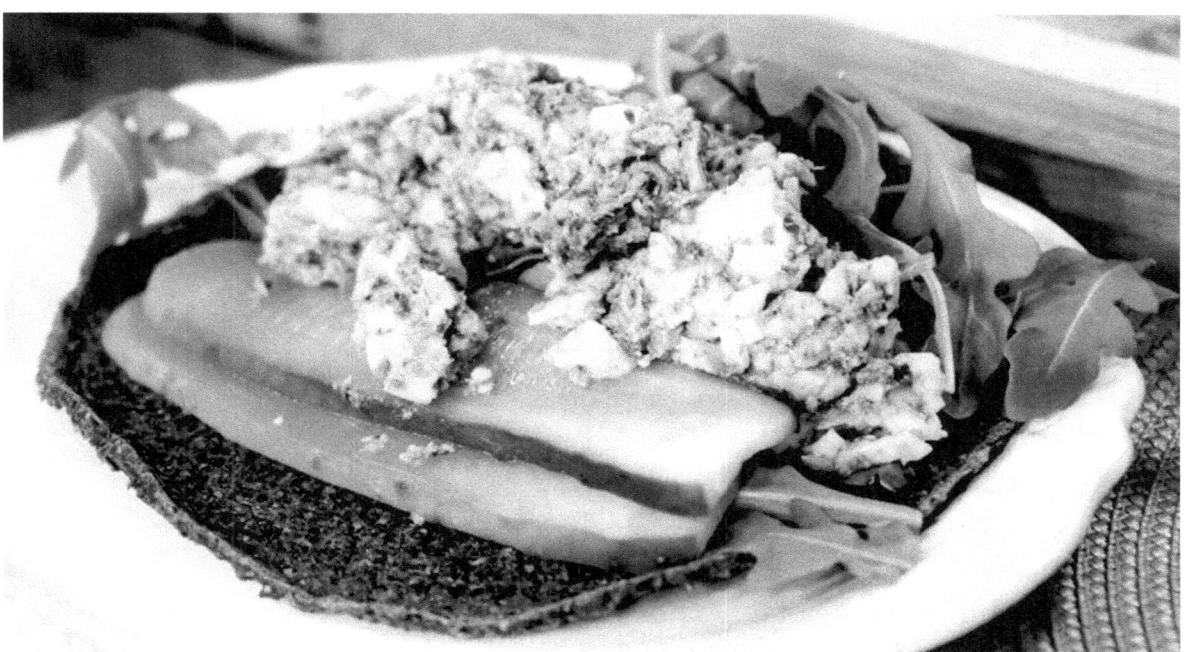

(**Freezer:** none / **Microwave:** none)

10. Barbecue Tofu sandwiches

(**Serves:** 6 / **Prep time:** 5 minutes / **Cooking time:** 10 minutes)

Nutritional Information (Per Serving)
Calories: 336
Carbohydrates: 47.1 g
Fat: 12.5 g
Protein: 9.4 g
Fiber: 2.1 g
Sodium: 945 mg

Ingredients
- Tofu (extra firm, 12 ounces)
- Bun of your choice (lettuce leaf, cabbage leaf)
- Vegetable oil (3 tbsp)
- Barbecue sauce (1 ½ c)
- Onion (sliced thin, 1)

Instructions
1. Make sure to get all of the water out of the tofu with a paper towel.
2. Slice it into pieces that are ¼ inch thick.
3. Take the vegetable oil and heat it up in the skillet.
4. Fry your tofu and put the onion in so that it can cook to your desired consistency.
5. Add the barbeque sauce and cook for ten minutes before serving.

(**Freezer:** None / **Microwave:** None)

11. Pesto pizza

(**Serves:** 6 / **Prep time:** 10 minutes / **Cooking time:** 10 minutes)

Nutritional Information (Per Serving)
Calories: 394
Fat: 19.9 g
Carbohydrates: 39.3 g
Protein: 17.3 g
Fiber: 3 g
Sodium: 937 mg

Ingredients
- Gluten free pizza crust (1)
- Feta cheese (crumbled, 1 c)
- Pesto (1/2 c)
- Artichoke hearts (drained, sliced, 4 oz.)
- Tomato (chopped, 1)
- Onion (chopped, ½)
- Bell pepper (green, chopped, ½)
- Black olives (chopped, drained, 2 oz.)

Instructions
1. Turn on your oven to 450 F
2. Cover the pizza crust with your pesto and your toppings
3. Bake for ten minutes or until your cheese has melted.

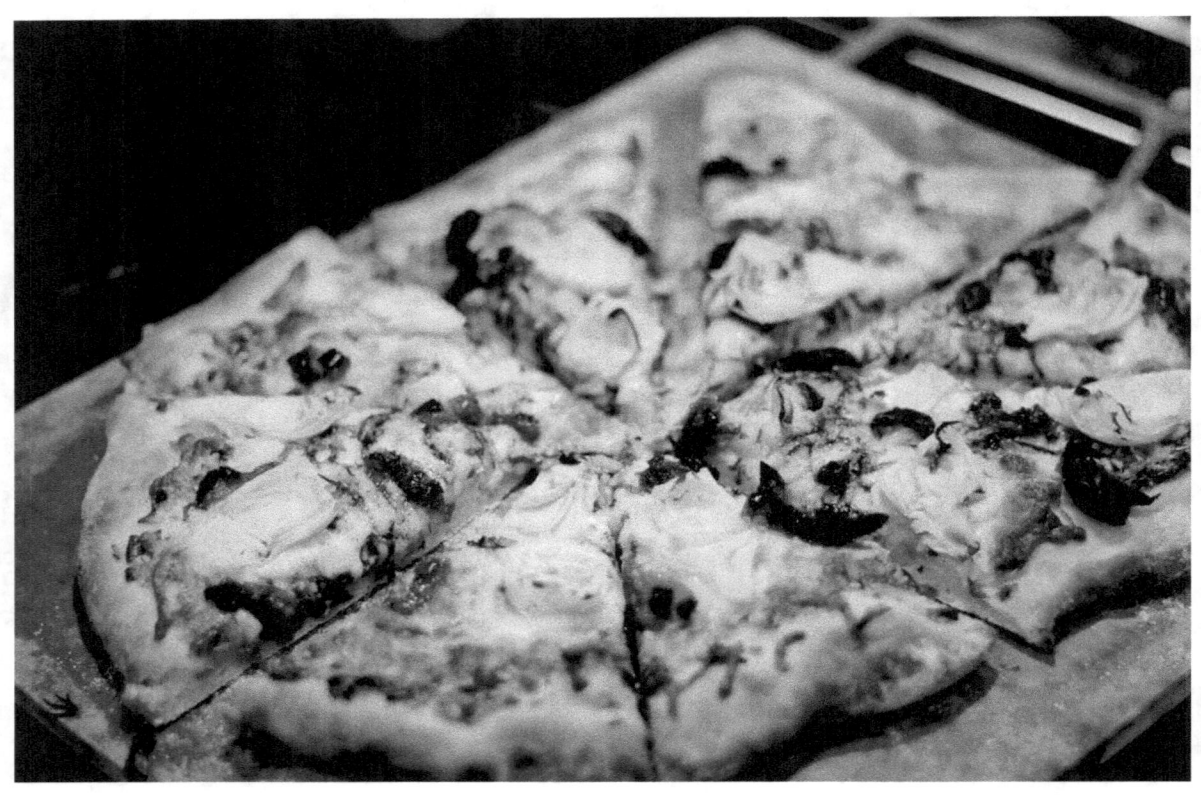

(**Freezer:** 1 month / **Microwave:** 30 seconds)

12. Grilled Portobello Mushrooms with Mashed Cannellini Beans and Harissa Sauce

(**Serves:** 4 / **Prep time:** 25 minutes / **Cooking time:** 13 minutes)

Nutritional Information (Per Serving)
Calories: 312
Protein: 17.1 g
Fat: 10 g
Carbohydrates: 44. 8 g
Sodium: 1192 mg
Fiber: 12.5 g

Ingredients

Harissa sauce
- Red pepper (1, roasted, minced, peeled)
- Cayenne pepper (1 pinch)
- Shallot (chopped, 2 tbsp)
- Black pepper (1 pinch)
- Garlic (minced, 1 tsp)
- Coriander (ground, 1 pinch)
- Olive oil (1 tsp)
- Red pepper flakes (1/4 tsp)
- Lime juice (1 tsp)
- Cilantro (fresh, minced, ½ tsp)
- Dijon mustard (3/4 tsp)

Mashed beans
- Black pepper (1/4 tsp)
- Cannellini beans (2 c)

- Truffle oil (2 tsp)
- Water (2 c)

Portobello mushrooms
- Black pepper (1/4 tsp)
- Portobello mushroom caps (4, large)
- Vegetable broth (1/2 c)
- Olive oil (4 tsp)

Instructions

1. Take the ingredients for the sauce and mix it in a bowl.
2. Then combine the beans with the water in a pan and cook on medium heat for five minutes before draining them.
3. Mix the beans with the truffle oil and the in the food processor until it is a smooth mixture.
4. Turn on the grill and oil the grates. Make sure you oil the mushroom caps as well.
5. Season the mushroom caps.
6. Grill four minutes a side.
7. Place ½ a cup of the puree in the mushroom cap topped with 2 tbsp of the sauce.

(**Freezer:** 3 months / **Microwave:** 1 minute)

13. Eggplant parmesan

(**Serves:** 10 / **Prep time:** 25 minutes / **Cooking time:** 35 minutes)

Nutritional Information (Per Serving)
Fat: 16 g
Carbohydrates: 62.1 g
Protein: 24.2 g
Calories: 487
Fiber: 8.8 g
Sodium: 1663 mg

Ingredients
- Basil (dried, ½ tsp)
- Eggplant (peeled, sliced, 3)
- Parmesan cheese (1/2 c)
- Mozzarella cheese (16 oz.)
- Eggs (2)
- Spaghetti sauce (6 c)
- Gluten-free flour

Instructions
1. Preheat oven to 350 F.
2. Dip eggplant into egg and then the flour.
3. Place in the pan and cook for five minutes.
4. Get another pan and cover with spaghetti sauce, top with eggplant sauces.
5. Sprinkle with cheese until there is nothing left. The top layer should be cheese.
6. Top off with basil.
7. Cook for 35 minutes.

(**Freezer:** 4 months / **Microwave:** 1 ½ minutes)

Fish and seafood

1. Czech Christmas fried fish

(**Serves:** 4 / **Prep time:** 15 minutes / **Cooking time:** 5 minutes)

Nutritional Information (Per Serving)
Protein: 35 g
Fat: 33.5 g
Carbohydrates: 6.9 g
Calories: 80
Fiber: 4.4 g
Sodium: 146 mg

Ingredients
- Ghee (1/4 cup)
- Carp, cod, or haddock fillets (4, skinless, wild caught)
- Flax meal (4 tablespoons)
- Caraway seeds (1 tablespoon, ground)
- Almond flour (1 cup)
- pepper (to taste)
- Coconut milk (1 tablespoon)
- Egg (1)

Instructions
1. In a mixing bowl, you need to mix your flax meal and almond flour together, so they are thoroughly incorporated.
2. Dry with a paper towel.
3. Season with your pepper, and caraway seeds.

4. In a different bowl, you will take your egg and crack it before beating the coconut milk in with it. You may want to add a pinch of just for some flavor.
5. Taking your dry fish fillets, you'll dip them into the egg mix before dropping them into the dry mix. Once they are coated, you will need to shake the extra coating off before setting aside.
6. Once all of the fillets have been covered, you'll heat up the ghee in a pan. Your breaded fish will be added in once the ghee has melted and you are going to fry the fish. Don't lay them on top of each other or they are not going to get done. It will take about three minutes a side or until the bottoms are crispy and have a golden-brown color. How long you have to cook the fish will depend on how thick the fillet is.
7. Now you will take your fish and serve it with your favorite side!

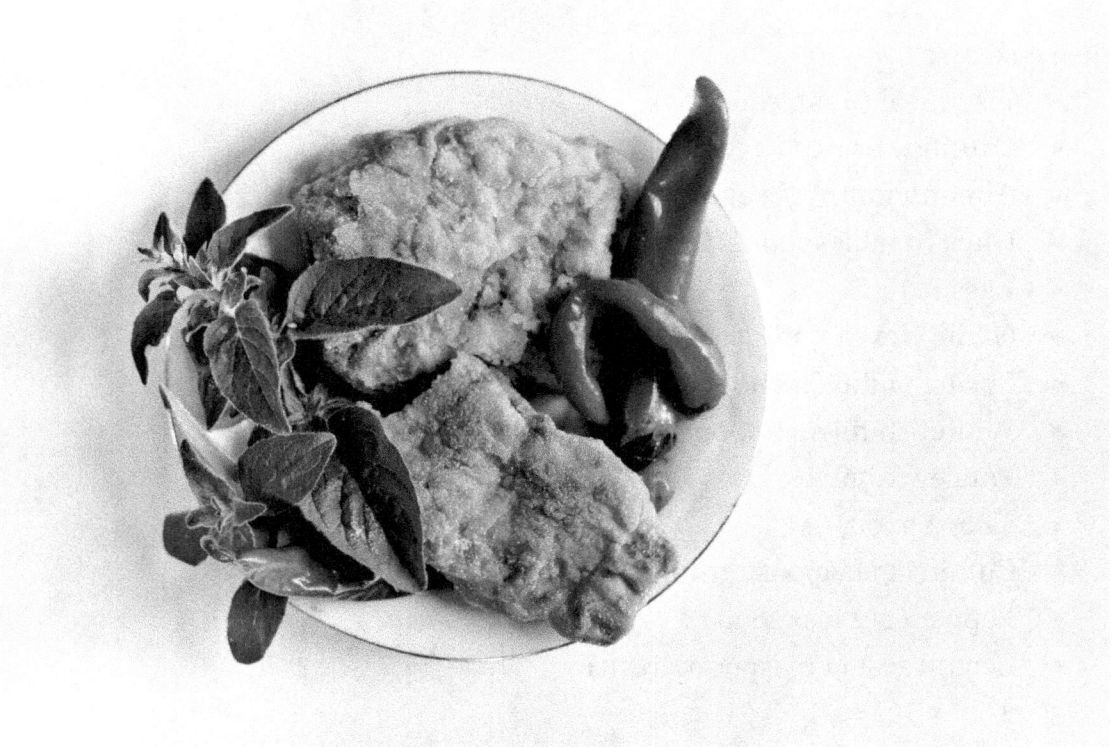

(**Freezer:** 1 month / **Microwave:** 3 ½ minutes)

2. Fish cakes with aioli

(**Serves:** 6 / **Prep time:** 30 minutes / **Cooking time:** 15 minutes)

Nutritional Information (Per Serving)
Calories: 460
Protein: 9.5g
Fat: 22.8g
Carbohydrates: 55.7g
Fiber: 3.2 g
Sodium: 97 mg

Ingredients

Fish cakes
- Flax meal (4 tablespoons)
- Cauliflower rice (2 cups)
- Almond flour (1/2 cup)
- Ghee (4 tablespoons)
- Eggs (2)
- Garlic clove (1, minced)
- Spring onion (1, chopped)
- Whitefish fillets (2 pounds, skinless, boneless)
- Parsley (2 tablespoons, fresh, chopped)
- (1 teaspoon)
- Cumin (1 teaspoon, ground)
- Pepper (1/2 teaspoon)
- Lemon zest (1 teaspoon, fresh)

Aioli
- Garlic cloves (2, minced)

- Mayonnaise (1/2 cup)

Instructions
1. Cook your cauliflower rice.
2. Cook your fish with some ghee in a skillet you'll cook for about three minutes without flipping them. Throw your rice, lemon zest, seasonings, egg, flour, and flax meal into a bowl together. Add in any pepper you have left. Combine thoroughly.
3. Take a ¼ measure cup and spoon the mixture from the bowl. Use the last of the ghee and heat up your frying pan. After it has gotten hot; lower the heat and put the patties in the pan. Allow them to cook until they are golden brown on each side.
4. Make your aioli by mixing your two ingredients together.

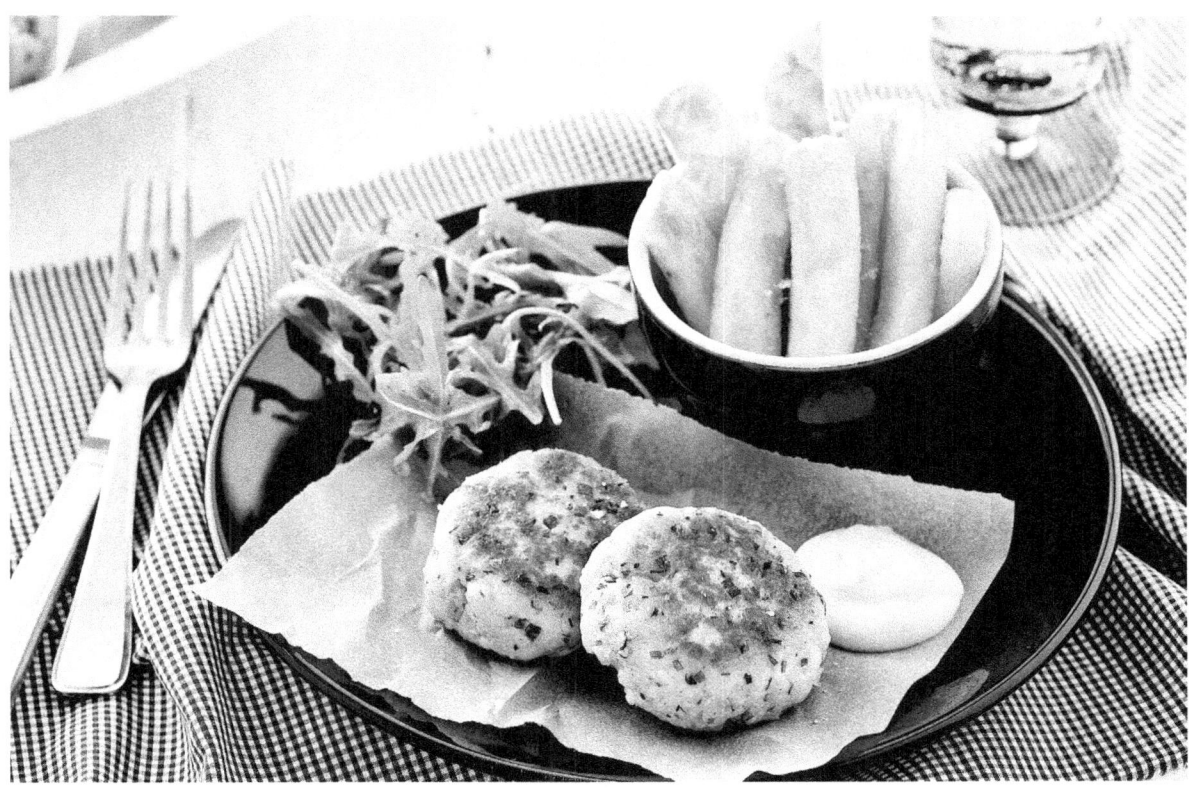

(**Freezer:** 3 months / **Microwave:** 20 seconds)

3. Grilled lobster

(**Serves:** 4 / **Prep time:** 15 minutes / **Cooking time:** 15 minutes)

Nutritional Information (Per Serving)
Protein: 44.3g
Calories: 742
Fat: 60.9 g
Carbohydrates: 4.3 g
Sodium: 958 mg
Fiber: 0.5 g

Ingredients
- Garlic cloves (2)
- Lobster tails (4)
- Butter (1/2 c)
- Seasonings (to taste)
- Olive oil (drizzle)

Instructions
1. Heat your grill to medium.
2. Remove the white part of the lobster.
3. Drizzle with olive oil and season.
4. Grill for seven minutes.
5. Flip and finish grilling this will be about five minutes.
6. As it cooks, melt the butter and add in the garlic.

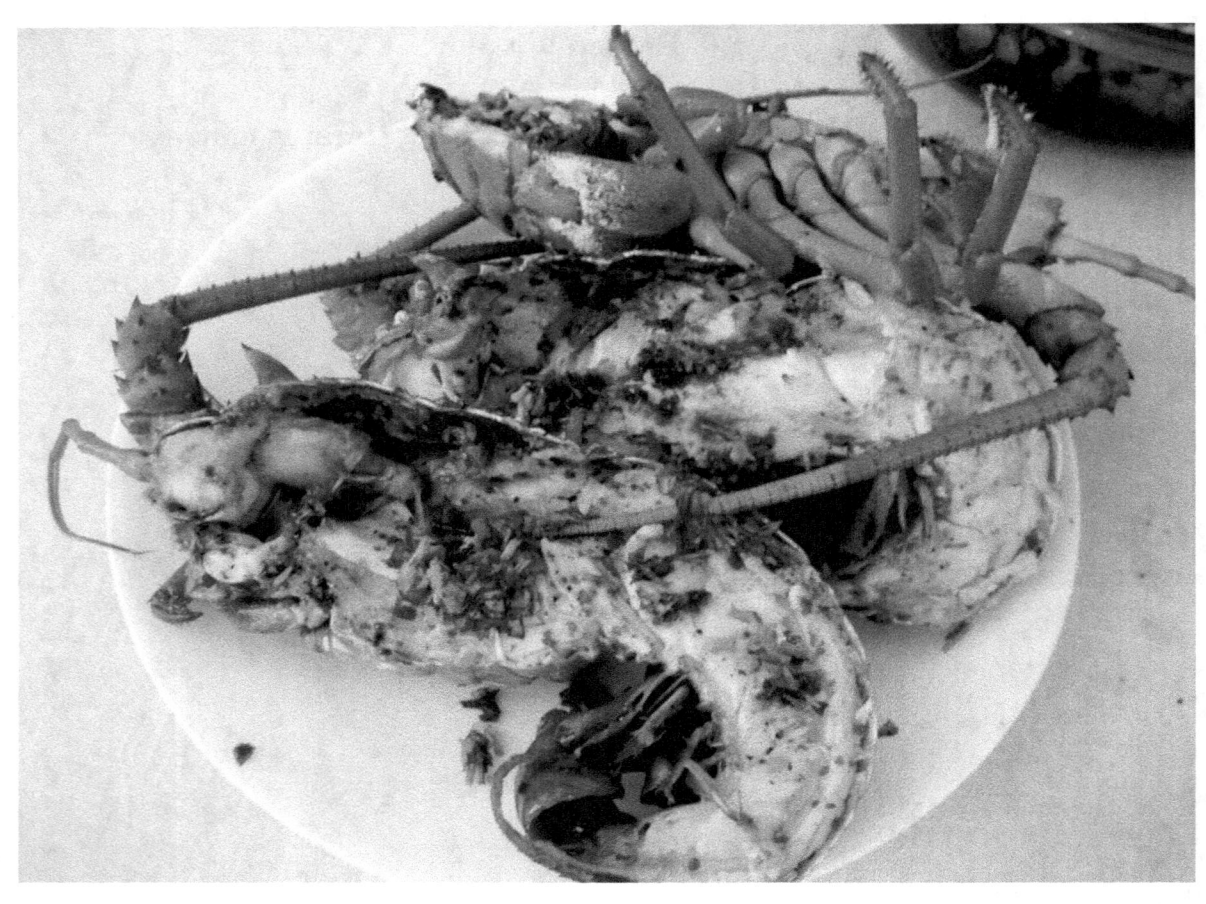

(**Freezer:** 2 months / **Microwave**: none)

4. Paleo sushi

(**Serves:** 2 / **Prep time:** 30 minutes / **Cooking time:** 5 minutes)

Nutritional Information (Per Serving)
Calories: 146.2
Fat: 8.6 g
Carbohydrates: 7.6 g
Protein: 11.1 g
Fiber: 5.5 g
Sodium: 877 mg

Ingredients
- Coconut aminos (handful)
- Nori (4 sheets)
- Coconut oil (1 tbsp)
- Avocados (5, mashed)
- Cucumber (1)
- Eggs (4, beaten)
- Salmon (8 oz., smoked)

Instructions
1. Cut the salmon up into strips.
2. Cut the cucumber up in slices.
3. Melt the coconut oil in a pan.
4. Dump in your eggs and allow for conforming to the pan to cook.
5. Put the shiny nori side down.
6. Spread out the avocado.
7. Put 2 salmon strips, 2 egg strips, 4 cucumber strips in the nori.
8. Roll and cut.

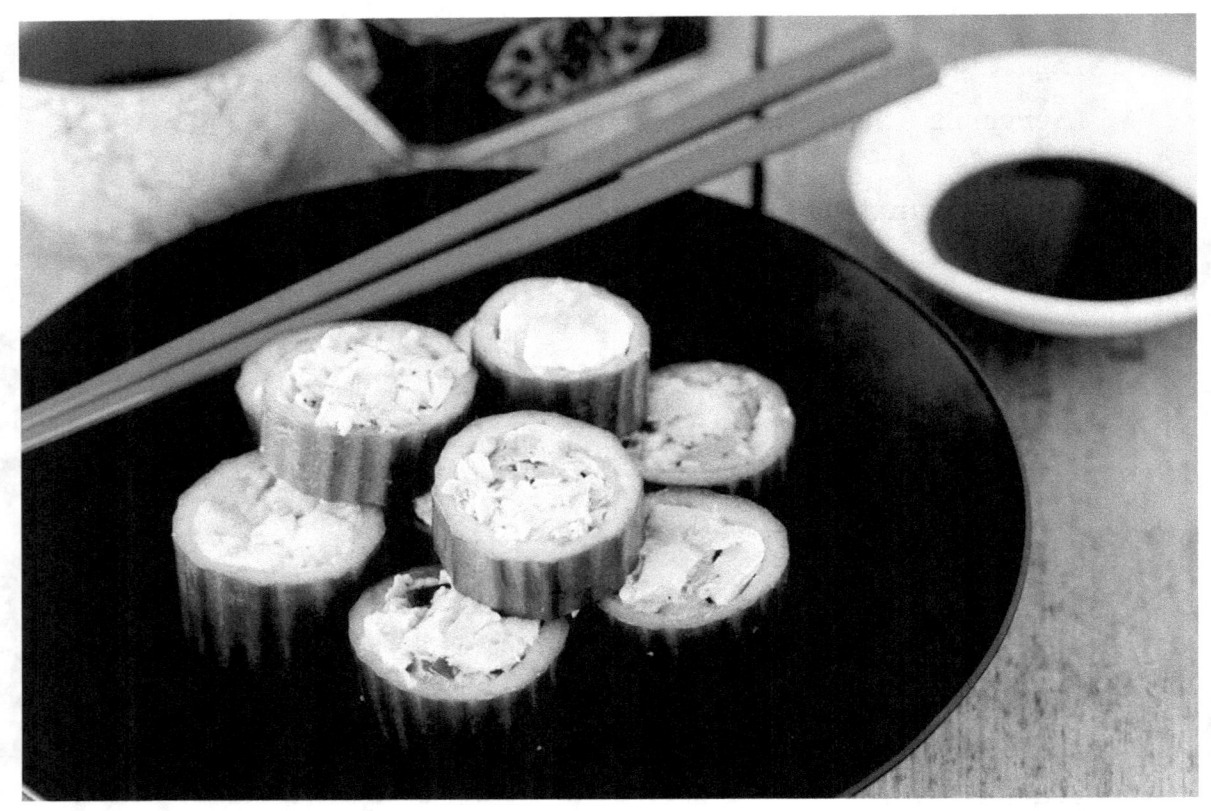

(**Freezer:** 1 month / **Microwave:** none)

5. Scrambled eggs with smoked salmon

(**Serves:** 2/ **Prep time:** 10 minutes / **Cooking time:** 8 minutes)

Nutritional Information (Per Serving)
Calories: 200.5
Fat: 13.3 g
Carbohydrates: 2.3 g
Protein: 16.7 g
Fiber: 1.9 g
Sodium: 562.9 mg

Ingredients
- Sea salt (to taste)
- Eggs (4)
- Cooking fat (a spoonful)
- Smoked salmon (4 slices, chopped)
- Chives (a few stalks, chopped)
- Coconut milk (2 tbsp)

Instructions
1. Whisk the eggs together with the milk and the chives.
2. Season your eggs to taste.
3. Take the fat and melt it in a skillet.
4. Dump your eggs into the skillet.
5. As the eggs are starting to settle, stir in the salmon and cook for two minutes.
6. Sprinkle with more chives and enjoy.

(**Freezer:** 1 month / **Microwave:** 1 ½ minutes)

6. Twisted tuna salad

(**Serves:** 7 / **Prep time:** 15 minutes / **Cooking time:** none)

Nutritional Information (Per Serving)
Calories: 464.6
Fat: 13.6 g
Carbohydrates: 27.9 g
Protein: 73.9 g
Fiber: 18.5 g
Sodium: 1347.1 mg

Ingredients
- Tuna (4 5 oz. cans, drained)
- Paleo may (1/2 c and an additional 2 tbsp)
- Carrot (1/2 c, chopped)
- Garlic clove (1, crushed)
- Celery (1/2 c, chopped)
- Scallions (4, chopped)
- Parsley (1/2 c, chopped)
- Onion (1/3 c, chopped)

Instructions
1. Take your tuna and drain it so that there is no water in it. Then, proceed to dump it into a bowl.
2. With your food processor, chop the celery, carrot, onion, parsley, and scallions.
3. Place in the bowl with the tuna and your garlic clove that you crushed as well as your mayo.
4. Mash up the tuna and thoroughly mix the ingredients together.
5. Chill and enjoy.

(**Freezer:** 1 month / **Microwave:** none)

7. Sunflower butter salmon with onions

(**Serves:** 1 / **Prep time:** 5 minutes / **Cooking time:** 20 minutes)

Nutritional Information (Per Serving)
Calories: 133
Protein: 21 g
Carbohydrates: 1 g
Fat: 4 g
Fiber: 0.8 g
Sodium: 562 mg

Ingredients
- Salmon fillet (4 ounces)
- Onion (1, sliced)
- Sunflower butter (1 tablespoon)
- Lemon juice (1/4 teaspoon)
- Vegetables of your choice (1/2 cup)

Instructions
1. Grill your salmon so that it is done to your liking.
2. Cook the onion in a skillet with olive oil until they reach a caramel color.
3. Take the onions off the heat and put them on your plate.
4. Heat the butter and lemon juice in your skillet but do not let it burn.
5. Place your salmon on your vegetables.
6. Drizzle with the butter mixture and serve.

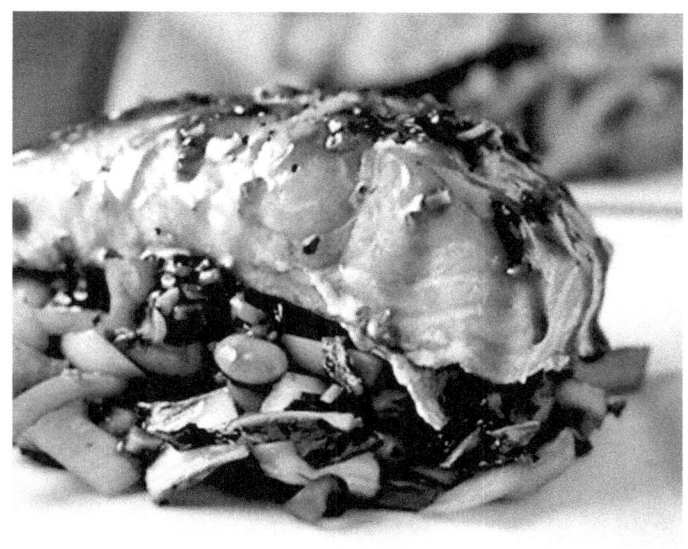

(**Freezer:** 1 month / **Microwave:** 3 minutes)

8. Macadamia crusted sea bass mango cream sauce

(**Serves:** 4 / **Prep time:** 20 minutes / **Cooking time:** 20 minutes)

Nutritional Information (Per Serving)
Calories: 423
Fat: 31.1 g
Protein: 24.2 g
Carbohydrates: 13.6 g
Fiber: 2.4 g
Sodium: 222 mg

Ingredients
- Mango (1, seeded, diced, peeled)
- Olive oil (1 tbsp, extra virgin)
- Heavy cream (1/2 c)
- Garlic cloves (2)
- Lemon juice (1 tsp)
- Black pepper (ground, to taste)
- Macadamia nuts (1/2 c)
- Seabass (1 lb.)
- Coconut flour (1/4 c)
- Red pepper flakes (a pinch)
- Olive oil (1 tsp)
- Black pepper (1/2 tsp)

Instructions
1. With the food processor, you'll put the nuts, flour, 1 tsp of olive oil, the pepper, and the red pepper flakes and process until it is smooth.
2. Make sure to turn your oven on 350 F.

3. In a saucepan, put the mango, lemon juice, and cream so that it can boil. Once it is cooked, it will need to simmer so it can thicken.
4. Season your fish as you heat a tablespoon of oil in a skillet with your garlic place your fish in the skillet and sear it on both sides.
5. Lastly, you'll move it to your oven and roast it until it is done cooking. After that, you'll cover it with your macadamia crust and cook it until it is browned.
6. Coat with cream sauce.

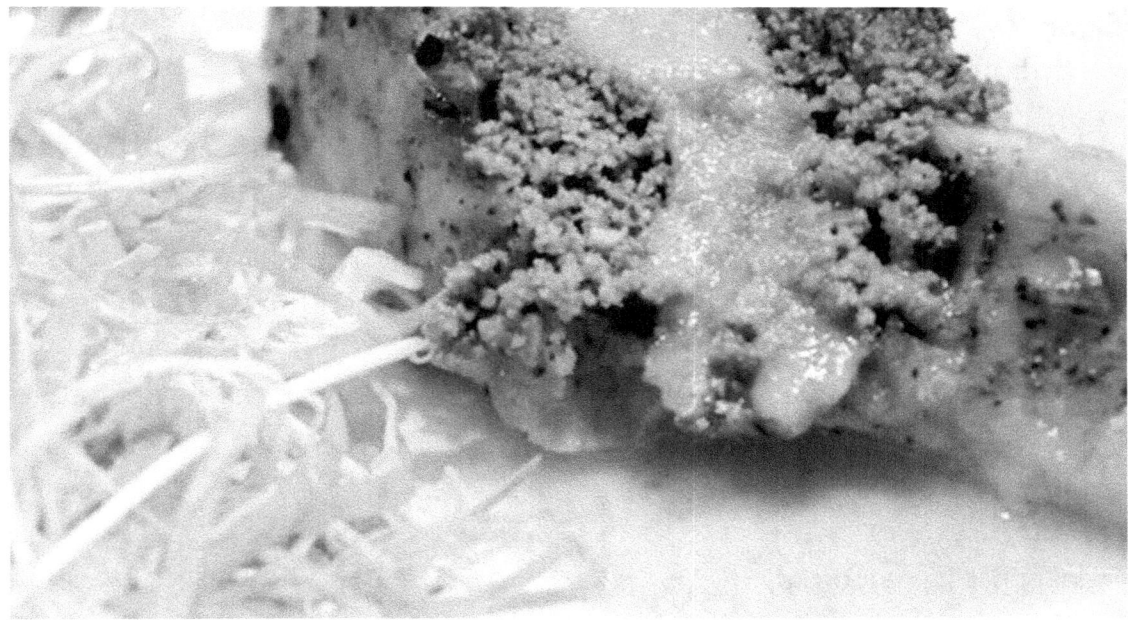

(**Freezer:** 1 month / **Microwave:** 4 minutes)

9. Peppered shrimp alfredo

(**Serves:** 6 / **Prep time:** 30 minutes / **Cooking time:** 20 minutes)

Nutritional Information (Per Serving)
Calories: 707
Protein: 28.4 g
Fat: 45 g
Fiber: 3.4 g
Sodium: 1034 mg
Carbohydrates: 50.6 g

Ingredients
- Penne pasta (gluten-free, 12 oz.)
- Parsley (1/4 c)
- Butter (1/4 c)
- Pepper (to taste)
- Olive oil (2 tbsp)
- Cayenne pepper (1 tsp)
- Garlic cloves (2)
- Cream (1/2 c)
- Pepper (1, red, diced)
- Romano cheese (1/2 c)
- Portobello mushroom (1/2 lb., diced)
- Alfredo sauce (15 oz.)
- Shrimp (1 lb., peeled, deveined)

Instructions
1. Boil water and insert your past so that it cooks to al dente.

2. Melt the butter with the olive oil before stirring in the onion and allowing it to cook until it is soft and translucent. Next stir in the garlic, pepper, and mushroom. It needs to cook on medium-high heat for around two minutes.
3. Stir in the shrimp and cook until firm. Now you will stir in the Alfredo sauce and the cheese. It will need to simmer and be stirred until it thickens.
4. After that, you'll season with the seasonings.

(**Freezer:** 3 months / **Microwave:** 2 ½ minutes)

10.   Salmon Cakes

(Serves: 4 / **Prep time:** 15 minutes / **Cooking time**: 10 minutes)

Nutritional Information (Per Serving)
Calories: 305
Fat: 14.6 g
Carbohydrates: 14.6 g
Protein: 30.9
Fiber: 2.8 g
Sodium: 846 mg

Ingredients
- Olive oil (1 tbsp)
- Red salmon (canned, skinned, deboned, drained, flaked, 14.75 oz.)
- Butter (1 tbsp)
- Eggs (2)
- Coconut flour (1 tbsp)
- Capers (1 tbsp, chopped)
- Crackers (12)
- Black pepper (1/2 tsp)
- Cayenne pepper (1/2 tsp)

Instructions
1. Stir together the lemon juice, capers, eggs, pepper, and cayenne pepper in a bowl.
2. Mix in the crackers with your hands and make sure to mix well.
3. Put the flour on a plate and divide out the salmon into four portions shaping them into patties. Sprinkle with flour.
4. Melt butter and oil in skillet and cook patties for about five minutes.

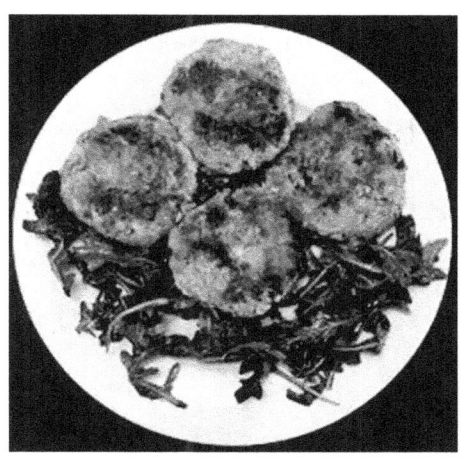

(**Freezer:** 2 months / **Microwave:** 90 seconds)

11. Grilled fish steaks

(**Serves:** 2 / **Prep time:** 10 minutes / **Cooking time:** 10 minutes)

Nutritional Information (Per Serving)
Calories: 554
Protein: 36.3 g
Fat: 43.7 g
Carbohydrates: 2.2 g
Fiber: 36.3 g
Sodium: 1259 mg

Ingredients
- Garlic clove (1)
- Halibut fillets (6 oz., 2)
- Olive oil (6 tbsp)
- Parsley (chopped, fresh, 1 tbsp)
- Basil (dried, 1 tsp)
- Lemon juice (fresh, 1 tbsp)
- Black pepper (1 tsp)

Instructions
1. Using a bowl combine the garlic, pepper, lemon juice, basil, parsley, and olive oil together.
2. Put the filets in a dish and marinade them with the mixture you just created. Allow to sit in the fridge for an hour, making sure to flip occasionally.
3. Turn on your grill and oil the grate. Make sure the grate is four inches from the heat source.
4. Drain the extra marinade off the filets and cook five minutes a side or until the fish is done. It should flake with a fork.

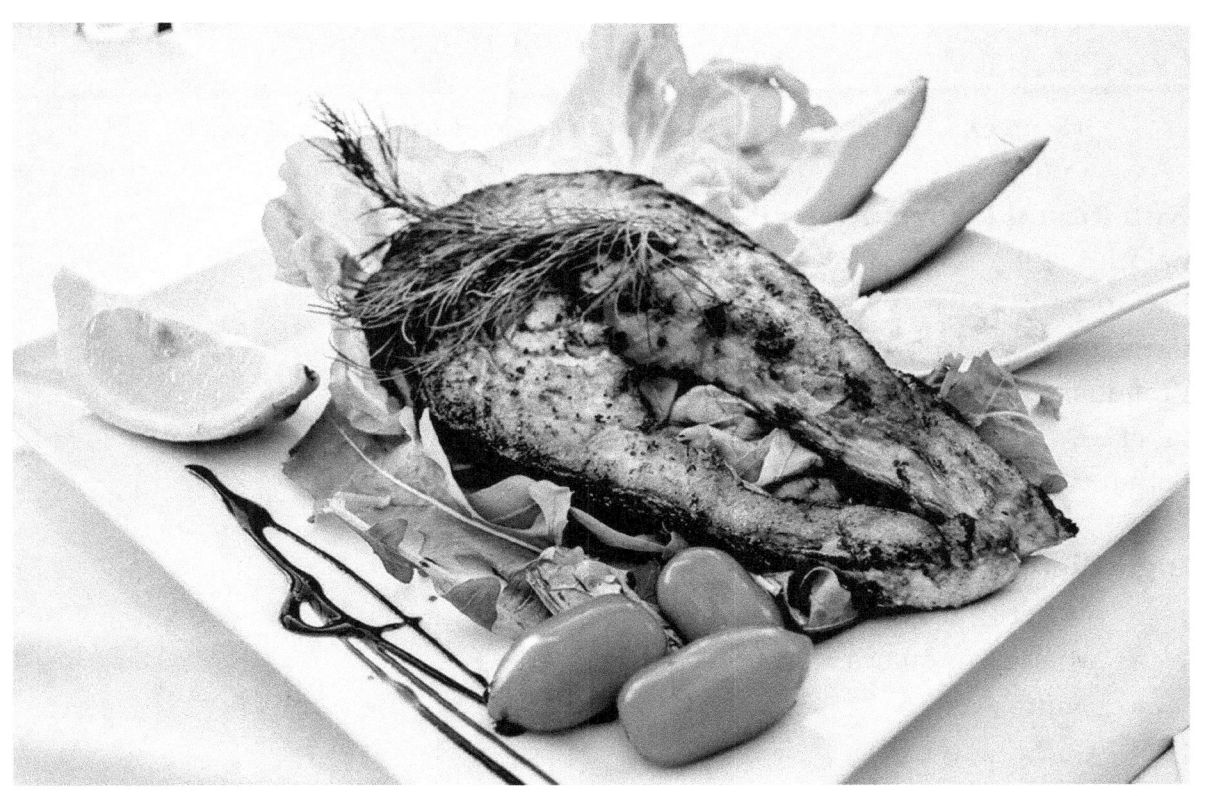

(**Freezer:** 7 months / **Microwave:** 3 minutes)

12. Mussels mariniere

(**Serves:** 4 / **Prep time:** 35 minutes / **Cooking time:** 15 minutes)

Nutritional Information (Per Serving)
Calories: 298
Fat: 10.1 g
Carbohydrates: 10.3 g
Proteins: 18.6 g
Fiber: 0.7 g
Sodium: 330 mg

Ingredients
- Butter (3 tbsp)
- Mussels (4 quarts, debearded, cleaned)
- White wine (2 c)
- Garlic cloves (2)
- Thyme (1/4 tsp, dried)
- Onion (1)
- Bay leaf (1)
- Parsley (chopped, 6 tbsp)

Instructions
1. Clean the mussels. Don't keep any mussels that have broken shells or cannot be closed.
2. Mix together the 4 tbsp of parsley, the bay leaf, onion, garlic, wine, thyme, and 2 tbsp of butter in a pot. Allow it to boil before you lower the heat allowing it to cook for 2 minutes. Throw in the mussels and cover it. You should let it cook until the shells pop open. Be careful not to overcook. Remove the mussels and put them in bowls.
3. Strain the liquid into the pot and then put it back.

4. Add in the rest of the butter and parsley allowing it to cook until the butter is melted. Then pour it over the mussels.

(**Freezer**: none / **Microwave:** none)

13. Penne with shrimp

(**Serves:** 8 / **Prep time:** 10 minutes / **Cooking time:** 25 minutes)

Nutritional Information (Per Serving)
Calories: 385
Fat: 8.5 g
Protein: 24.5 g
Carbohydrates: 48.5 g
Fiber: 3.5 g
Sodium: 399 mg

Ingredients
1. Parmesan cheese (1 cup)
2. Penne pasta (16 ounces)
3. Shrimp (1 pound)
4. Red onion (1/4 cup)
5. Diced tomatoes (2 14.5 ounce cans)
6. Chopped garlic (1 tablespoon)
7. White wine (1/4 cup)

Instructions
1. Take a large pot and boil water in the pan. Add in the pasta and allow it to cook for ten minutes or until it is al dente before you drain it.
2. In a skillet heat your oil and stir in onion and garlic. The onion needs to be tender before you mix in the tomatoes and wine before you cook it for another ten minutes.
3. Throw the shrimp into the skillet and continue to cook until the shrimp is opaque until you put the pasta in before topping with parmesan cheese.

(**Freezer:** 2 months / **Microwave:** 3 minutes)

Poultry

1. Chicken Salad Lettuce Wraps

(**Serves**: 4 / **Prep time:** 10 minutes / **Cooking time:** 30 minutes)

Nutritional Information (Per Serving)
Calories: 250
Fat: 15 g
Carbohydrate: 10 g
Protein: 20 g
Fiber: 3.2 g
Sodium: 1893 mg

Ingredients

Chicken
- Olive oil (1 tablespoon)
- Chicken thighs (1 pound, boneless)
- Garlic powder (1/4 teaspoon)
- (1/2 teaspoon)
- Pepper (1/2 teaspoon)

Salad
- Romaine lettuce leaves (10 leaves)
- Celery (1 cup, diced)
- (to taste)
- Parsley (1 tablespoon, chopped)
- Mayonnaise (1/2 cup)
- Pepper (to taste)

Instructions
1. Turn your oven on to 390F.
2. Take a bowl and mix your chicken in with some pepper, olive oil, and garlic powder.
3. You will then place your chicken on a cookie sheet and cook it for about thirty minutes.
4. Once it is cooked, you will need to take it out of the oven and allow it to cool for about twenty minutes.
5. Take that chicken and put it in a bowl with the celery, mayonnaise, and parsley. You will need to mix everything together so that the chicken is coated with the seasoning.

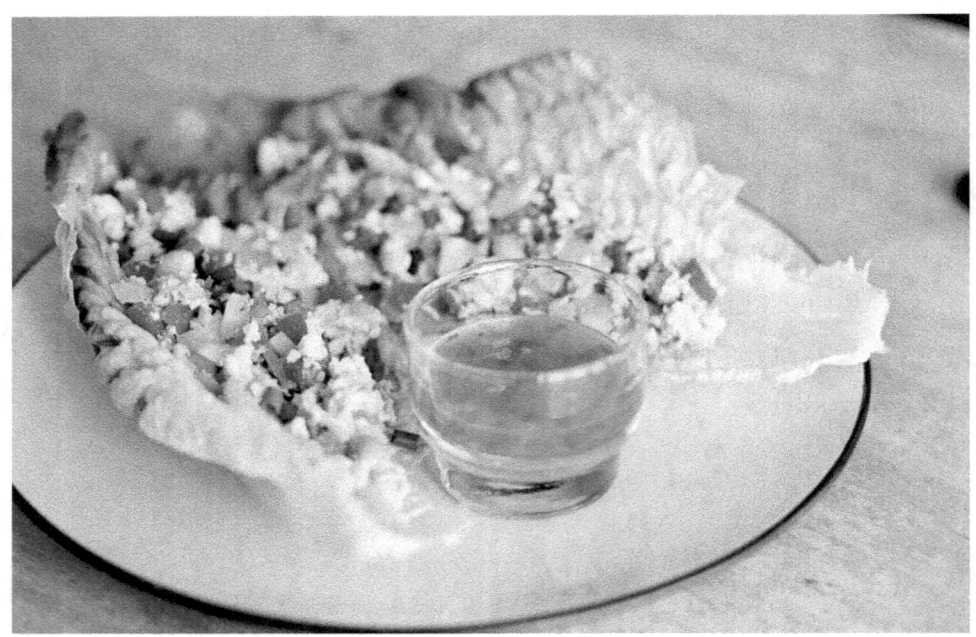

(**Freezer:** 5 months / **Microwave:** none)

2. Chili lime crispy chicken wings

(**Serves:** 8 / **Prep time:** 20 minutes / **Cooking time:** 1 hour 10 minutes)

Nutritional Information (Per Serving)
Calories: 132.5
Fat: 5.9 g
Carbohydrates: 5.0 g
Protein: 15.4 g
Fiber: 0.5 g
Sodium: 644.4 mg

Ingredients
- Ghee (2 tablespoons, melted)
- Chicken wings (4.4 pounds, cut at the joint)
- (1 teaspoon)
- Baking powder (2 tablespoons, gluten-free)

Chili lime sticky sauce
- Fish sauce (1 tablespoon)
- Sukrin gold syrup (1/4 cup)
- Coconut aminos (1/4 cup)
- Lime juice (1/4 cup, fresh)
- Sriracha (1 tablespoon)
- Garlic cloves (4, minced)
- Ginger (1 tablespoon, grated)

Instructions
1. Turn your oven on to 250 F and move your racks so that they are in the middle of the oven. Pick a pan that will be thick enough to collect all of the fat off of the chicken wings while they are baking. Take aluminum foil and

line the pan so that it is easy for you to clean. Take a drying rack and place it on top of the foil

2. Anything that is remaining will go into a large bowl and be tossed with the baking powder.
3. After coating the wings, you'll place them on the rack with the skin up. Now take a cooking brush and brush your melted ghee over the meat before cooking them for thirty minutes.
4. After thirty minutes, move the rack up and turn your oven up to 425 F. allowing them to cook for another fifty minutes. At the halfway point, you will need to rotate your tray so that the wings cook evenly. Make your chili lime sticky sauce. All of the ingredients need to be placed into a pan and combined as they are brought to a boil on medium-low heat. It should be allowed to cook for about ten minutes or until the sauce thickens.

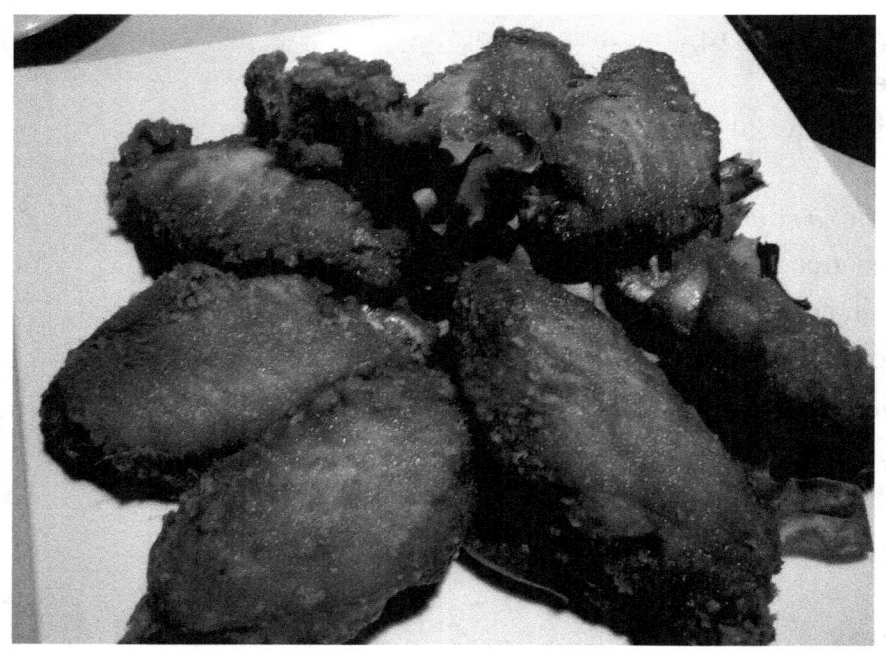

(**Freezer:** 4 months / **Microwave:** 4 minutes)

3. Chicken fajitas

(**Serves:** 6 / **Prep time:** 20 minutes / **Cooking time:** 40 minutes)

Nutritional Information (Per Serving)

Calories: 0.5
Fat: 0 g
Carbohydrate: 0 g
Protein: 0.1 g
Fiber: 0 g
Sodium: 3.5 mg

Ingredients

Chicken

- Ghee (2 tablespoons)
- Chicken breasts (1 pound, skinless, boneless)
- Lemon juice (2 tablespoons)
- Garlic cloves (2, minced)
- Olive oil (1/4 cup)
- Herbs (1 teaspoon, dried oregano, paprika, ground cumin)
- (1 teaspoon)
- Chipotle chili powder (1/2 teaspoon)

Vegetables

- Ghee (2 tablespoons)
- Onion (1, sliced)
- Pepper (1, sliced, orange or yellow)
- Red pepper (1, sliced)
- Green pepper (1, sliced)

Other
- Keto tortillas (6)

Instructions
1. Cut your chicken into strips and place in a bowl. Add in all the spices including the lemon juice and olive oil.
2. Coat the chicken on all sides and allow to marinate either thirty minutes in the fridge.
3. Peel your onion and slice it. Slice the peppers as well. In a dish, grease it down and heat it up over medium-high heat. After the pan gets hot, you will toss in your vegetables.
4. Cook until they are tender. Stir so that they do not burn. Do not touch the heat, just re-grease the pan and cook your chicken until it is light brown
5. Place your peppers back in the pan and cook for thirty seconds.

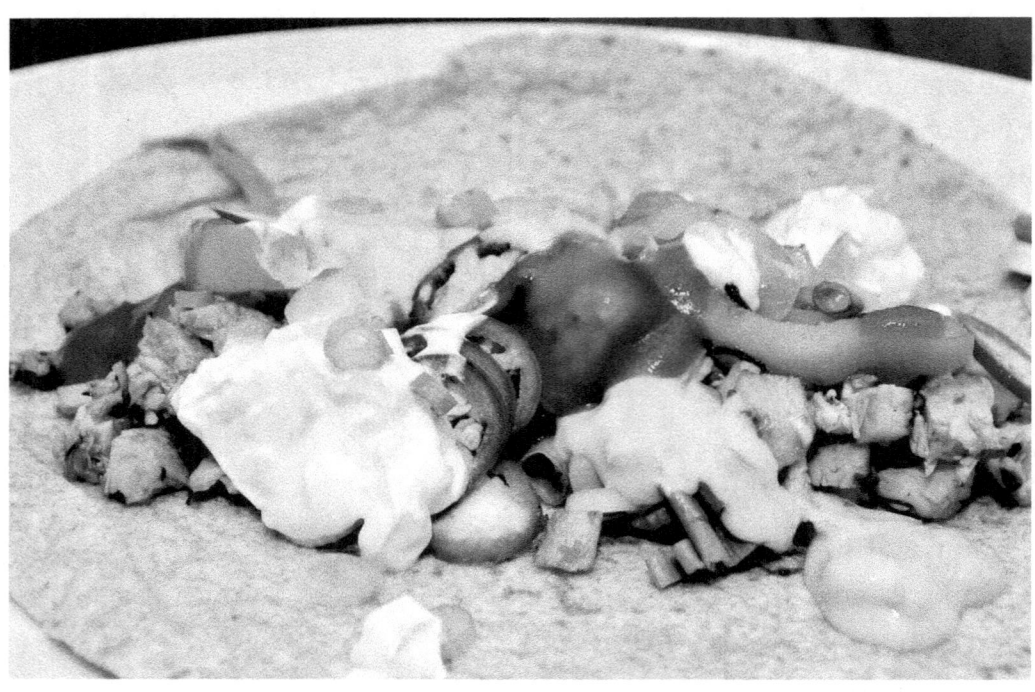

(**Freezer:** 4 months / **Microwave**: 1 ½ minutes)

4. Low carb chicken fricassee

(**Serves:** 4 / **Prep time:** 20 minutes / **Cooking time:** 10 minutes)

Nutritional Information (Per Serving)
Calories: 219.5
Fat: 6.6 g
Carbohydrate 9.2 g
Protein: 27.8 g
Sodium: 410.1 mg
Fiber: 1.8 g

Ingredients
- Pepper (to taste)
- Chicken thighs (1 pound, sliced)
- Cauliflower rice (4 cups, uncooked)
- Fresh herbs (2 tablespoons, your choice)
- Ghee (4 tablespoons)
- Egg yolks (4)
- Onion (1, diced)
- Coconut milk (1 cup)
- Garlic cloves (2, minced)
- Paprika (1 teaspoon)
- Celery (1, sliced)
- Bay leaf (1, crumbled)
- Mushroom (1 cup, sliced)
- White wine (1/2 cup, dry)
- Lemon juice (2 tablespoons, fresh)
- Chicken stock (1/2 cup)

Instructions
1. Cut your chicken and season it with salt. Put in a skillet that is greased with ghee and toss the chicken in, so it can cook till it is completely brown.
2. After this is done, use a slotted spoon and move the chicken to a bowl.
3. Put more ghee in your skillet and add in the onion and garlic. Cook until fragrant. Then add in the mushroom and celery. Cook for a minute.
4. Dump in the stock and lemon juice along with the wine and bay leaf. Also, put the paprika in and allow it to boil.
5. Whisk the milk with the egg yolks and drizzle into the pan as it is cooking. Allow it to thicken before adding in the herbs that you chose to use.
6. Place your chicken back into your casserole and mix for about two minutes.
7. In another pot make your cauli-rice.

(**Freezer:** 1 month / **Microwave:** 3 minutes)

5. Grilled veggie and grilled chicken salads with tomato vinaigrette

(**Serves:** 2 / **Prep time:** 10 minutes / **Cooking time:** 20 minutes)

Nutritional Information (Per Serving)
Calories: 261
Fat: 21.4 g
Protein: 3.5 g
Carbohydrates: 16.4 g
Fiber: 2.4 g
Sodium: 747 mg

Ingredients

Chicken
- Chicken breast (1 lb.)
- Rosemary (1 tsp)
- Olive oil (1 tbsp)

Veggies
- Zucchini (1)
- Olive oil (1 tbsp)
- Squash (1, yellow)
- Onion (1)
- Cherry tomatoes (2 c, fresh)
- Pepper (1, red)

Instructions
1. Toss the olive oil and spices on the chicken breasts.
2. Cut the veggies and toss in olive oil.
3. Heat the grill up.

4. Put the chicken on one side and vegetables on tin foil on the opposite side.
5. Cook for about eight minutes.
6. Flip and cook until thoroughly cooked, and veggies are soft.

(Freezer: 2 months / **Microwave:** 3 minutes)

6. Spicy Indian chicken stir fry

(**Serves:** 4 / **Prep time:** 2 hours and 20 minutes / **Cooking time:** 25 minutes)

Nutritional Information (Per Serving)
Fat: 9 g
Protein: 59 g
Carbohydrates: 24 g
Fiber: 2.3 g
Sodium: 606 mg

Ingredients

- Red chili paste (2 tbsp)
- Chicken breasts (4, stripped)
- Cumin (1/2 tsp)
- Carrots (4, sliced)
- Chili powder (1 tsp)
- Onion (1, minced)
- Chili powder (1 tsp)
- Bell peppers (2, chopped)
- Ginger paste (1 tbsp)
- Green chilies (2, sliced)
- Garlic paste (1 tbsp)

Marinade
- Egg (1, beaten)
- Ginger (2 tsp, minced)
- Tapioca starch (2 tbsp)
- Garlic cloves (2, minced)
- Cumin powder (1 ½ tsp)

- Turmeric powder (2 tsp)
- Coriander powder (1 tsp)
- Red chili powder (1 tsp)

Instructions
1. Combine all the marinade ingredients.
2. Mix the chicken in until coated well and put in the fridge for up to two hours.
3. Melt the fat in a pan.
4. Brown the chicken.
5. Remove and set aside.
6. Add garlic, ginger, cumin and chili powder cook for about three minutes.
7. Toss in rest of the vegetables and allow them to soften.
8. Put the chicken back in the pan and cook for ten minutes.

(**Freezer:** 3 weeks / **Microwave:** 3 minutes)

7. Cracklin' chicken

(Serves: 4 / **Prep time:** 10 minutes / **Cooking time:** 15 minutes)

Nutritional Information (Per Serving)
Sodium: 340 mg
Fiber: 0 g
Calories: 80
Fat: 6.0 g
Carbohydrates: 0 g
Protein: 7 g

Ingredients
- Seasonings of your choice (to taste)
- chicken thighs (4 lbs., skin on, bone in)
- Ghee (2 tsp)

Instructions
1. Take a pair of sharp kitchen shears and cut out the bone from the chicken thigh. Try not to cut through the meat and stay as close to the bone as you can.
2. Remove the bone, joint, and cartilage.
3. Use a meat pounder and flatten out the chicken.
4. Take a skillet and put it on medium high.
5. Melt the ghee in the pan and set your chicken in the pan skin down.
6. Season the side that is up with your favorite seasonings.
7. Do not touch and allow to fry for about 10 minutes.
8. Flip the chicken after ten minutes and cook for another three minutes.
9. Move to a wire rack and allow to dry for about five minutes.

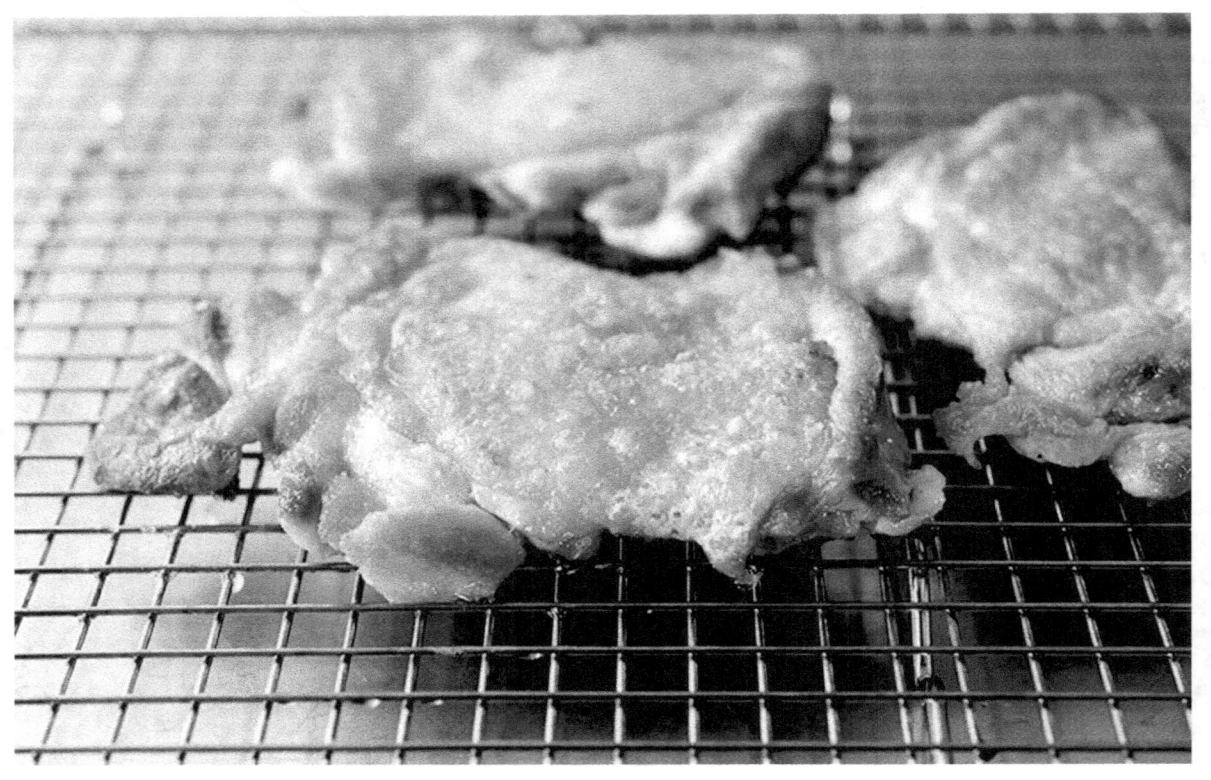

(**Freezer:** 4 months / **Microwave:** 4 minutes)

8. Grilled chicken breasts with zucchini

(**Serves:** 4 / **Prep time:** 15 minutes / **Cooking time:** 35 minutes)

Nutritional Information (Per Serving)
Fat: 24 g
Protein: 62 g
Carbohydrates: 10 g
Fiber: 0.1 g
Sodium: 104 mg

Ingredients

Chicken:
- Chicken breast (4, bone in, skin on)
- Parsley (1 tsp, dried)
- Cumin seeds (2 tbsp)
- Oregano (1 tsp, dried)
- Garlic cloves (2, minced)
- Paprika (1 tbsp)

Zucchini
- Zucchini (4, sliced)
- Olive oil (drizzle)
- Lemon zest (1 lemon)
- Garlic powder (1/4 tsp)
- Oregano (1/2 tsp, dried)

Instructions
1. Put the grill on medium-high heat.
2. Mix seeds, cloves, paprika, parsley, and oregano in a bowl.

3. Rub chicken in mix.
4. Put on the rack, skin down and cook for about thirty-five minutes, flip about every five minutes.
5. Mix the zucchini with anything you have left over.
6. Grill for three minutes a side.

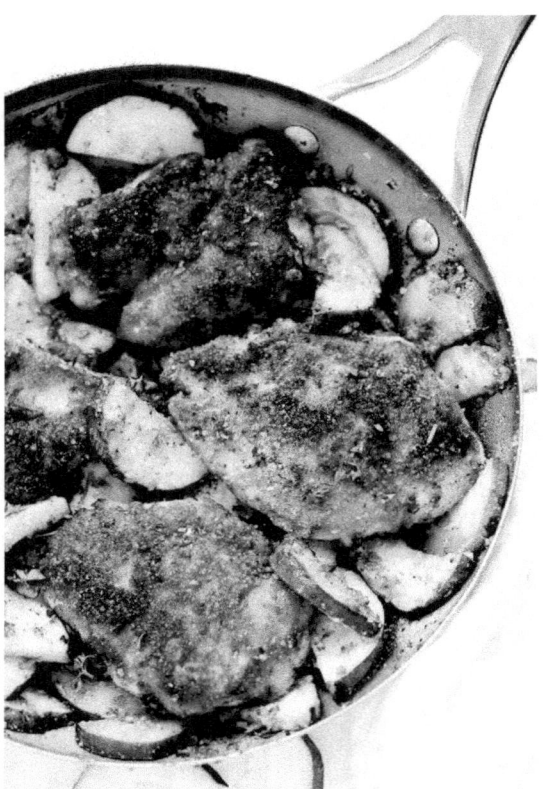

(**Freezer:** 1 month / **Microwave:** 2 minutes)

9. Keto harissa chicken skewers

(**Serves:** 4 / **Prep time:** 10 minutes / **Cooking time:** 110 minutes)

Nutritional Information (Per Serving)
Calories: 321
Fat: 14.3 g
Protein: 27.9 g
Carbohydrates: 23.1 g
Sodium: 49 mg
Fiber: 1.5 g

Ingredients

- Olive oil (2 tablespoons and another 4 tablespoons)
- Chicken breasts (1 pound)
- Harissa paste (1/3 cup)

Instructions

1. Cut the chicken into pieces.
2. Put in a bowl with the paste and the 2 tablespoons of oil. Cover and let sit in the fridge for two hours. Once ready, place on skewers.
3. Cook in an oven preheated to 440 F and cook for up to fifteen minutes.
4. Drizzle with the remaining oil and serve.

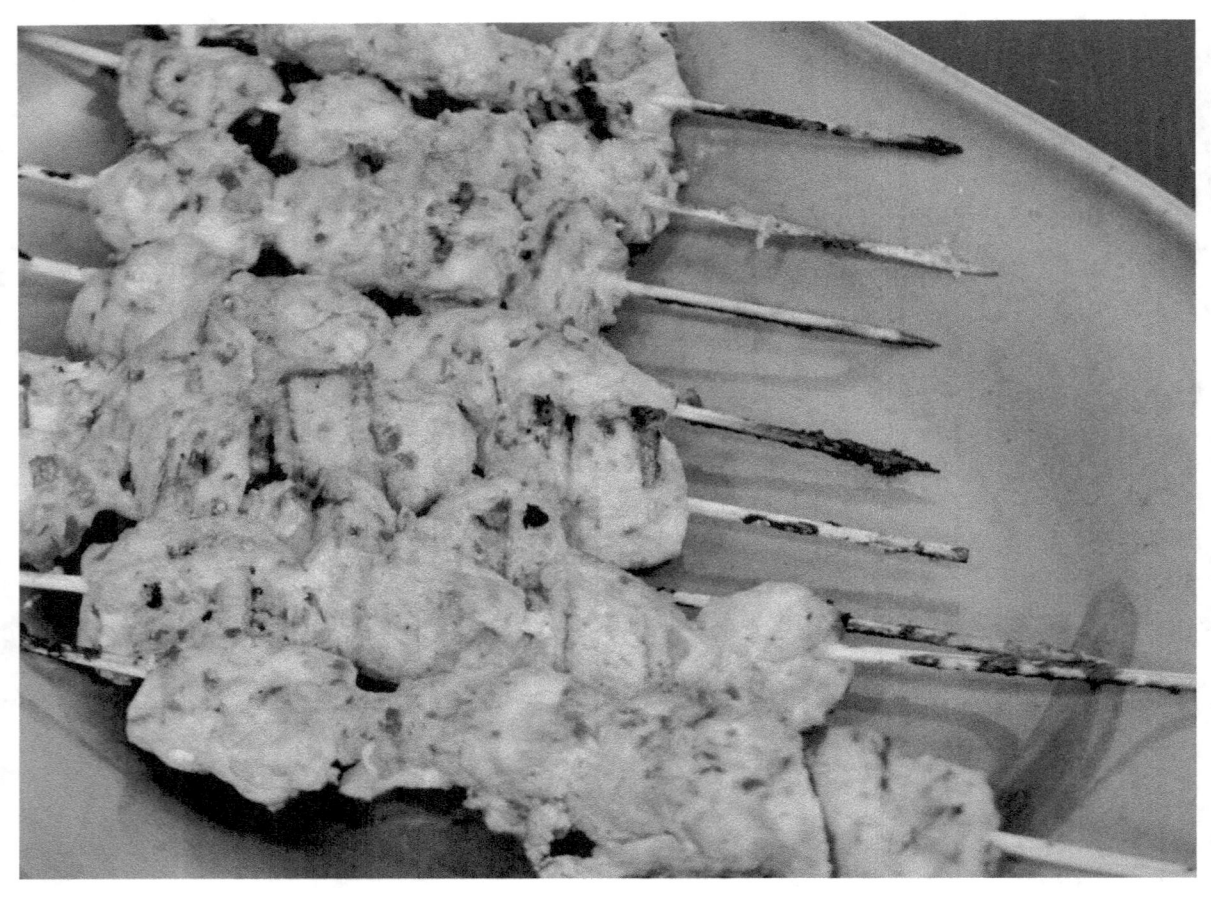

(**Freezer:** 1 month / **Microwave:** 4 minutes)

10. Chicken with cauliflower and olives

(**Serves:** 4 / **Prep time:** 1 hour / **Cooking time**: 15 minutes)

Nutritional Information (Per Serving)
Calories: 520.9
Fat: 40.5 g
Carbohydrate: 7.9 g
Protein: 31. 9
Fiber: 4.2 g
Sodium: 585 mg

Ingredients

- garlic cloves (5, sliced)
- chicken breasts (1 pound, skinless, boneless)
- Kalamata olives (1 cup, pitted)
- Thyme (1 sprig, fresh)
- Lemon juice (1/4 cup, raw)
- Cauliflower (1, cut into florets)
- Lemon zest (1 tablespoon)
- Shallot (1, chopped)
- Pepper (1 teaspoon)
- Olive oil (3 tablespoons)

Instructions

1. Rinse off the chicken and dry.
2. Put the thyme on the bottom of a baking pan and put the chicken over it.
3. Cover with cauliflower.
4. Mix the shallot, oil, and seasonings in a bowl.

5. Dump over the chicken and cauliflower.
6. Set in the fridge overnight.
7. Turn on the oven to 400 F and cook for forty-five minutes or until the cauliflower is brown.

(**Freezer:** 2 months / **Microwave:** 3 ½ minutes)

11. Chicken tomato and green bean curry

(Serves: 6 / **Prep time:** 15 minutes / **Cooking time:** 30 minutes)

Nutritional Information (Per Serving)
Calories: 104
Fat: 6.6 g
Carbohydrates: 11.2 g
Protein: 2.6 g
Sodium: 10 mg
Fiber: 3.9 g

Ingredients

- Coconut oil (2 tbsp)
- Green beans (1 lb., fresh, trimmed)
- Onion (1, chopped)
- Water or broth (1/2 c)
- Garlic cloves (6, chopped)
- Chicken thighs (2 ½ lbs., skinless, boneless)
- Cumin (1 ½ tbsp.)
- Tomatoes (28 oz., crushed)
- Chili powder (1 ½ tbsp.)
- Cayenne pepper (1/4 tsp)
- Turmeric (1 tsp)

Instructions
1. Use the food processor to chop the onion.
2. Chop the garlic separately.
3. Mix the chili powder, cumin, cayenne, and turmeric together.
4. Cut the chicken into 1-inch strips.

5. Wash the green beans and chop into pieces.
6. Put a pot over medium-high heat.
7. Mix in ghee.
8. Add in onion and cook for ten minutes.
9. Add in garlic and cook for another 2 minutes.
10. Toss in the other spices and continuously stir.
11. Mix in the crushed tomatoes and cook for 5 minutes.
12. Stir in chicken and liquid you chose.
13. Boil before covering and reducing heat. Allow to cook for ten minutes.
14. Check to see if the chicken is done.
15. Add in green beans and cook for another five minutes.

(**Freezer:** 4 months / **Microwave:** 2 ½ minutes)

Meat

1. Mug muffin with beef, mushrooms, and cheese

(**Serves:** 2 / **Prep time:** 10 minutes / **Cooking time**: 15 minutes)

Nutritional Information (Per Serving)
399 Milligrams Potassium
124 Milligrams Magnesium
434 Kilocalories
37.2 Grams Fat
18.7 Grams Protein
6.5 Grams Fiber
8.9 Grams Carbs
230.4 milligrams Sodium

Ingredients
- Flour (almond, 0.9 ounces)
- Water (2 tablespoons)
- Flax meal (1.3 ounces)
- Coconut milk or cream (2 tablespoons)
- Baking soda (0.25 teaspoons)
- Egg (1)
- Parsley (chopped)
- Basil (chopped)
- Ground beef (32 grams)
- Cheddar cheese (.5 cup)
- Mushrooms (.9 ounces)

Instructions

1. Cook the meat until there is no pink.
2. Get rid of the liquid except for one tablespoon.
3. Cut the mushrooms up and cook them for about five minutes or until they are browned.
4. Take all of your dry ingredients and mix them in a bowl.
5. With a fork, mix in the cream, water, and egg until it is combined well.
6. Combine the beef and mushrooms to the mixture.
7. Divide up into two mugs and add in any extras you may want.
8. Microwave for ninety seconds.
9. Let sit for five minutes.
10. Enjoy!

Note: if you don't have a microwave, cook it in the oven for fifteen minutes at 175 C (350 F)

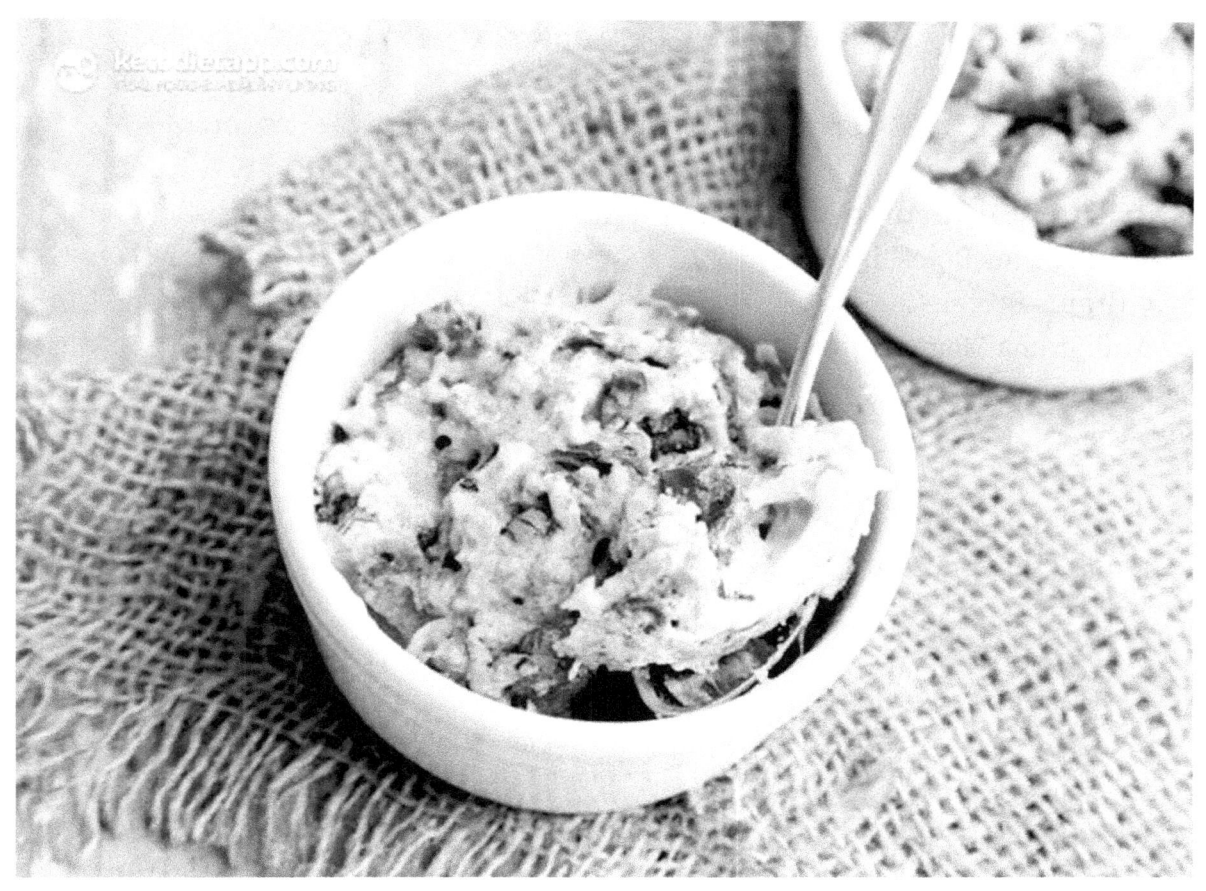

(**Freezer:** 3 months / **Microwave:** 90 seconds)

2. Beef and egg stuffed pattypan squash

(**Serves:** 4 / **Prep time:** 20 minutes / **Cooking time:** 25 minutes)

Nutritional Information (Per Serving)
546 Milligrams Potassium
19.9 Grams Protein
62 Milligrams Magnesium
31.4 Grams Fat
400 Kilocalories
10.7 Grams Carbs
2.7 Grams Fiber
224 milligrams sodium

Ingredients
- Pattypan squash (4)
- Eggs (4)
- Garlic (cloves, 2)
- Parmesan cheese (grated, 3 ounces)
- Onion (white, 1)
- Ground beef (1 cup)
- Ghee (1.9 ounces)

Instructions
1. Turn the oven on to 175 C (350 F).
2. Cut the top off the squash and remove the guts.
3. Keep the guts in a bowl for later.
4. Cover the top of the squash with ghee that has been melted
5. Put on a cookie sheet and cook for twenty minutes. They should be fork tender when they come out.
6. Put the onion and garlic in a pan with the ghee that is left over and cook until they are brown. This will be about five minutes.

7. Cook the ground beef until it is brown. Be sure to stir the mixture so that it does not burn.
8. Take all the seeds from the guts that you took out of the squash. The soft seeds are okay to keep if you want so that you can roast them later on.
9. After your beef has browned. Mix the squash guts in and cook for about five minutes.
10. If the parmesan is not already grated, go ahead and grate it.
11. Place the cheese in the pan and season to taste. Mix everything together until it is combined thoroughly.
12. Place the mixture into the squash and crack an egg on the inside of the squash to cover the beef mixture.
13. Cook for about twenty minutes or until the egg is done but the yolk is runny still.

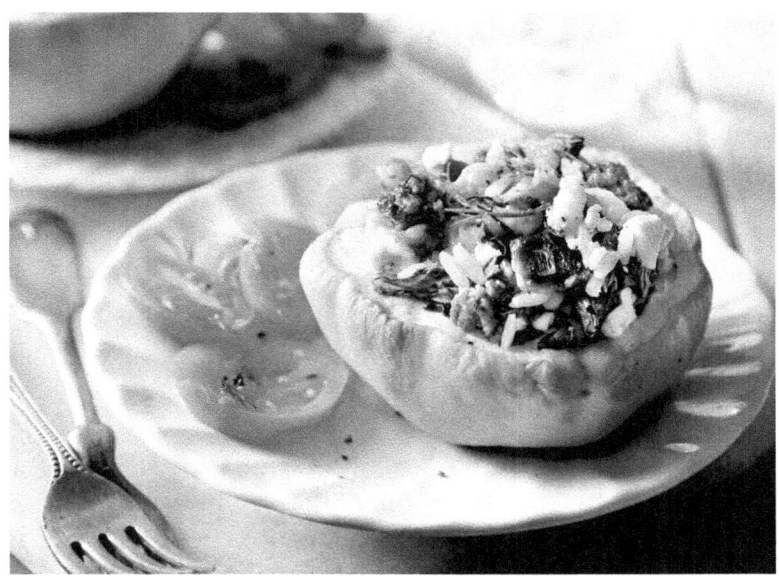

(**Freezer:** 2 months / **Microwave:** 2 ½ minutes)

3. Grain Free Breakfast Taco Pie Filling

(**Serves:** 8 / **Prep time:** 30 minutes / **Cooking time:** 45 minutes)

Nutritional Information (Per Serving)
Calories: 524.8
Fat: 30.1 g
Sodium: 894.7 mg
Carbohydrate: 42.5 g
Protein: 20 g

Ingredients
- Mango salsa (optional)
- Ground beef (grass fed, 340.194 grams or ¾ pounds)
- Baking soda (0.3 tablespoons, 1 teaspoon)
- Taco seasoning (9 teaspoons, 3 tablespoons)
- Coconut oil (0.3 tablespoons, 1 teaspoon)
- Onion (white 0.5)
- Cilantro (to taste)
- Bell pepper (red, 0.5)
- Eggs (grass fed, 8)

Instructions
1. Cook the meat in the oil.
2. Once browned, add in seasonings to taste.
3. Remove juice.
4. Using the same pan, sauté onion and bell pepper together with juice you drained off the meat.
5. Mix eggs, baking soda, and cilantro together.
6. Add more cilantro to onion and bell pepper.
7. Place in meat mix in pie crust.
8. Add onion and bell pepper.

9. Top off with eggs.
10. Cook for 45 minutes at 176.6 C or 350 F.
11. Serve with salsa if so desired but enjoy!

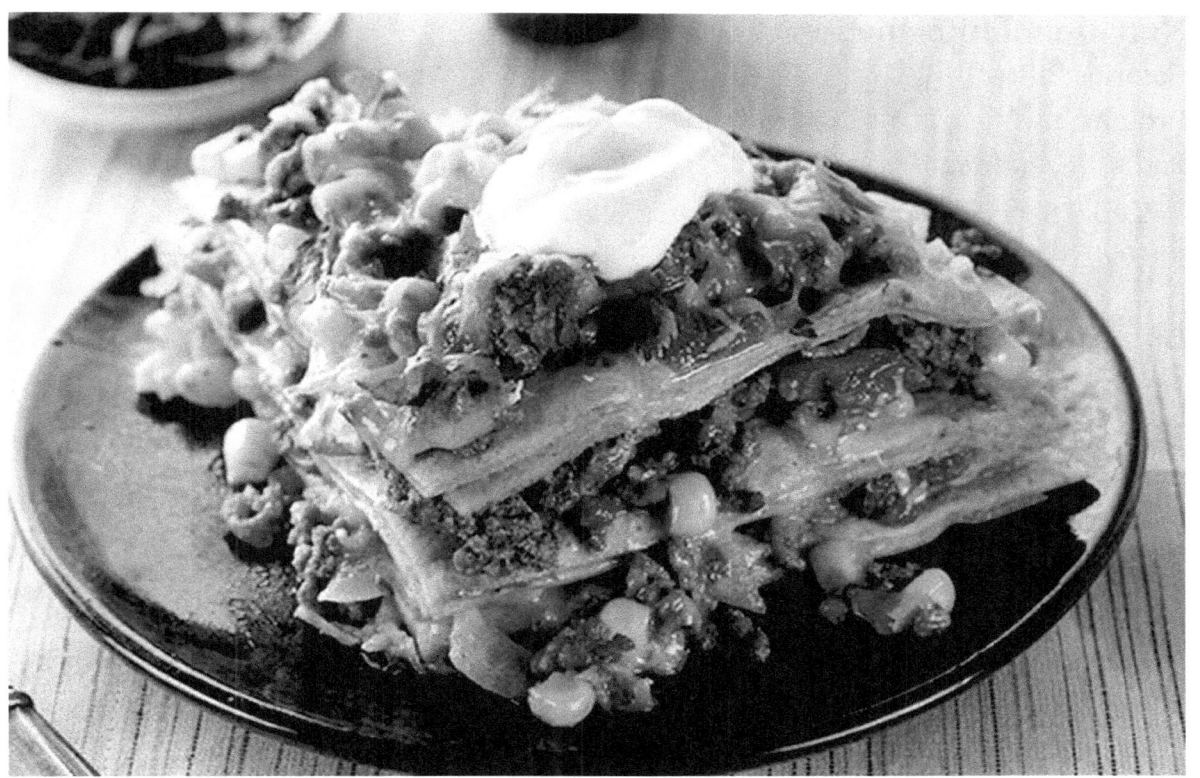

(**Freezer:** 1 ½ months / **Microwave:** 3 ½ minutes)

4. Spaghetti squash lasagna

(**Serves:** 12 / **Prep time:** 10 minutes / **Cooking time:** 80 minutes)

Nutritional Information (Per Serving)
Calories: 280
Protein: 14.1 g
Sodium: 1294 mg
Fat: 15.9 g
Carbohydrates: 24.5 g

Ingredients
- Ground beef (48 ounces, 3 pounds)
- Mozzarella cheese (30 slices)
- Spaghetti squash (2 large)
- Marinara sauce (1133.98 grams, 40 ounces)
- Ricotta cheese (whole milk, 907.18 grams, 32 ounces)

Instructions
1. Turn on the oven to 190.5 C (375 F).
2. Cut the squash in half and place face down in a pan of water.
3. Cook for 45 minutes until the skin can be peeled off.
4. Brown the meat in a skillet.
5. Place meat in a saucepan and mix with marinara.
6. Once the squash is done, cut out squash guts.
7. Put lasagna in a pan that is greased (squash, beef, mozzarella, ricotta).
8. Do this until there is nothing left.
9. Cook for another 35 minutes or until bubbles.

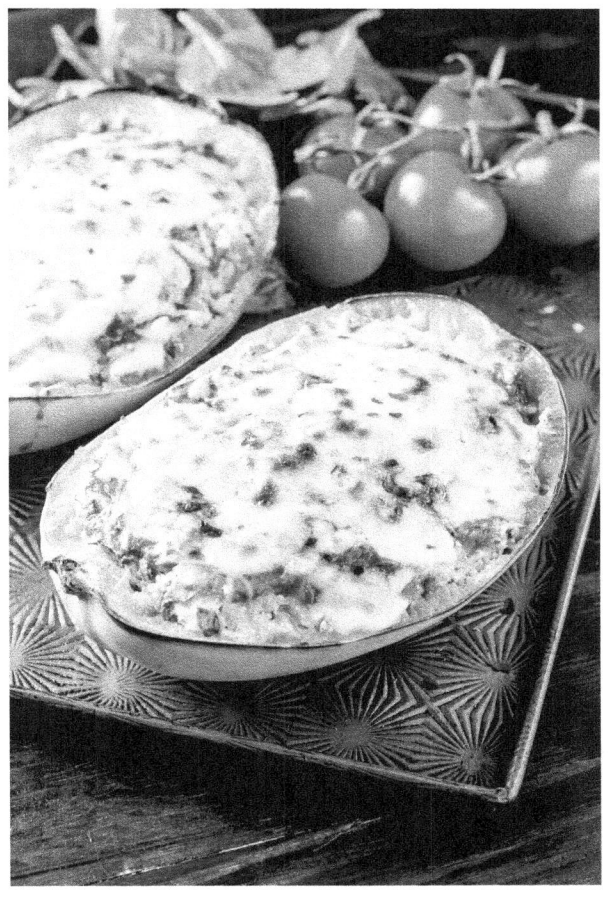

(**Freezer:** 6 months / **Microwave:** 4 minutes, 15 seconds)

5. Mexican spinach casserole

(**Serves:** 12 / **Prep time:** 15 minutes / **Cooking time:** 45 minutes)

Nutritional Information (Per Serving)
- 11 Carbohydrates
- 403 Calories
- 26 Grams Protein
- 27 Grams Fat
- 3 Grams Fiber
- 845 grams sodium

Ingredients
- Spinach (drained, 2.5 cups)
- Ground beef (32 ounces)
- Jalapenos (optional)
- Rotel (drained, 2 cans)
- Taco seasoning (4 teaspoons)
- Mozzarella cheese (shredded, 1 cup)
- Cream cheese (2 cups)
- Onion (medium, 1)
- Sour cream (10 tablespoons)
- Pepper (green, 1)

Instructions
1. Cook onions and pepper after dicing them. They should be translucent.
2. Add in jalapenos if desired.
3. Place in a bowl.
4. Cook spinach until thawed if frozen, get rid of as much moisture from spinach as possible.
5. Place in prep bowl with vegetables.

6. Cook meat until brown.
7. Cook in taco seasoning.
8. Move to bowl.
9. Add in rotel after draining.
10. Add in sour cream, cream cheese, and mozzarella and mix thoroughly.
11. Place in a large pan (9 x 13).
12. Cook for 40 minutes at 176.6 C (350 F).

(**Freezer:** 2 months / **Microwave:** 3 minutes)

6. Taco cups

(**Serves:** 5 / **Prep time:** 10 minutes / **Cooking time:** 15 times)

Nutritional Information (Per Serving)
- 9.7 Grams Carbohydrates
- 511 Calories
- 38.4 Grams Protein
- 35.6 Grams Fat
- 284 milligrams sodium
- 1.5 grams fiber

Ingredients
Fathead nacho cups
- Chili powder (to taste)
- Mozzarella (shredded, 6 Ounces)
- Coriander powder (1 teaspoon)
- Flour (almond, 3 ounces)
- Cumin powder (1 teaspoon)
- Cream cheese (2 tablespoons)
- Egg (1)

Beef mix
- Tomato paste (1 tablespoon)
- Onion (sliced, 1)
- Chili powder (.5 teaspoon)
- Tomatoes (canned, sliced, 14 ounces)

Sides (optional)
- Sour cream
- Salad
- Avocado
- Guacamole

- Mozzarella (shredded)
- Salsa

Instructions

Meat mix
1. Fry the onion until they become clear.
2. Add in broken up meat and cook until thoroughly brown.
3. Mix in the spices, canned tomatoes, and tomato paste.
4. Cook for fifteen minutes without a cover.

Taco cups
1. Combine cheese, flour in a bowl.
2. Throw in cream cheese and microwave for a minute.
3. Stir and cook for another thirty seconds.
4. Pull out, stir, and add spices and egg to mix.
5. Place on a cookie sheet between two pieces of parchment paper.
6. Create circles with the dough using a cookie cutter or glass.
7. Move each cup to a muffin tin.
8. Cook for fifteen minutes at 220 C (425 F).
9. Pull out of the tin and bake for 2 more minutes on parchment paper.

Put it together
1. Put on a plate and create your cup.
2. Enjoy with your favorite sides.

Note: You can also use coconut flour

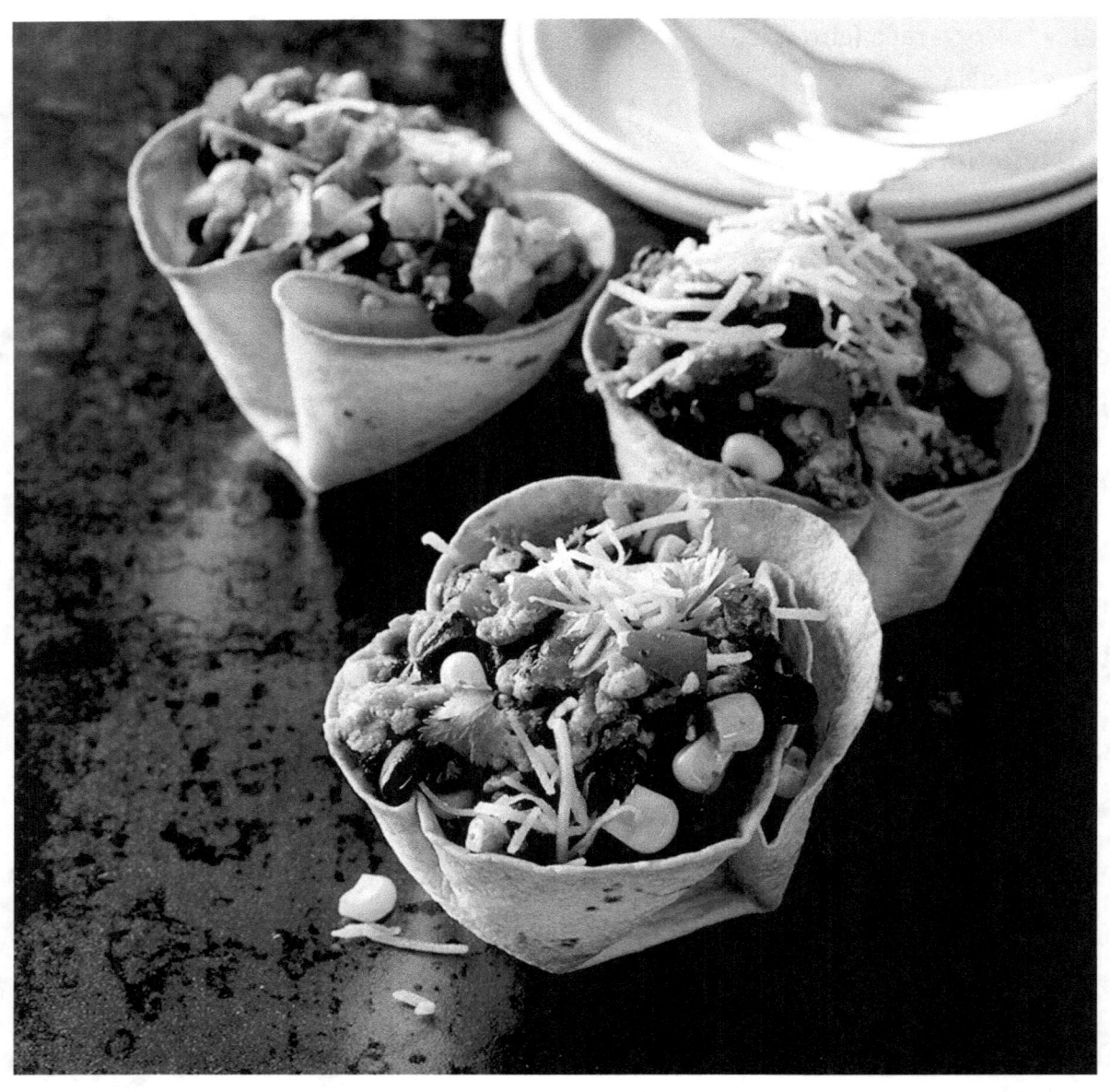

(**Freeze:** 5 months / **Microwave:** 2 ½ minutes)

7. Cheesy beef casserole

(Serves: 8 / **Prep time:** 15 minutes / **Cooking time:** 25 minutes)

Nutritional Information (Per Serving)
- 7 Carbohydrates
- 351 Calories
- 34 Grams Protein
- 17 Grams Fat
- 1 Grams Fiber
- 269.4 milligrams sodium

Ingredients
- Green onions (4 stalks)
- Ground beef (16 ounces)
- Salsa (green, 2 cups)
- Sour cream (8 ounces)
- Taco seasoning (4 teaspoons)
- Monterey Jack cheese (1 cup)
- Green chilies (diced, .5 cups)

Instructions
1. Cut up ground beef.
2. Cook until there is no pink left.
3. Drain liquid.
4. Add in taco seasoning.
5. Move into a pan that has been greased.
6. Mix salsa, chili, and sour cream and put over beef.
7. Cook for around twenty-five minutes at 176.6 C (350 F).
8. Add cheese before cooking for another five minutes.
9. Cool and place green onions on top.

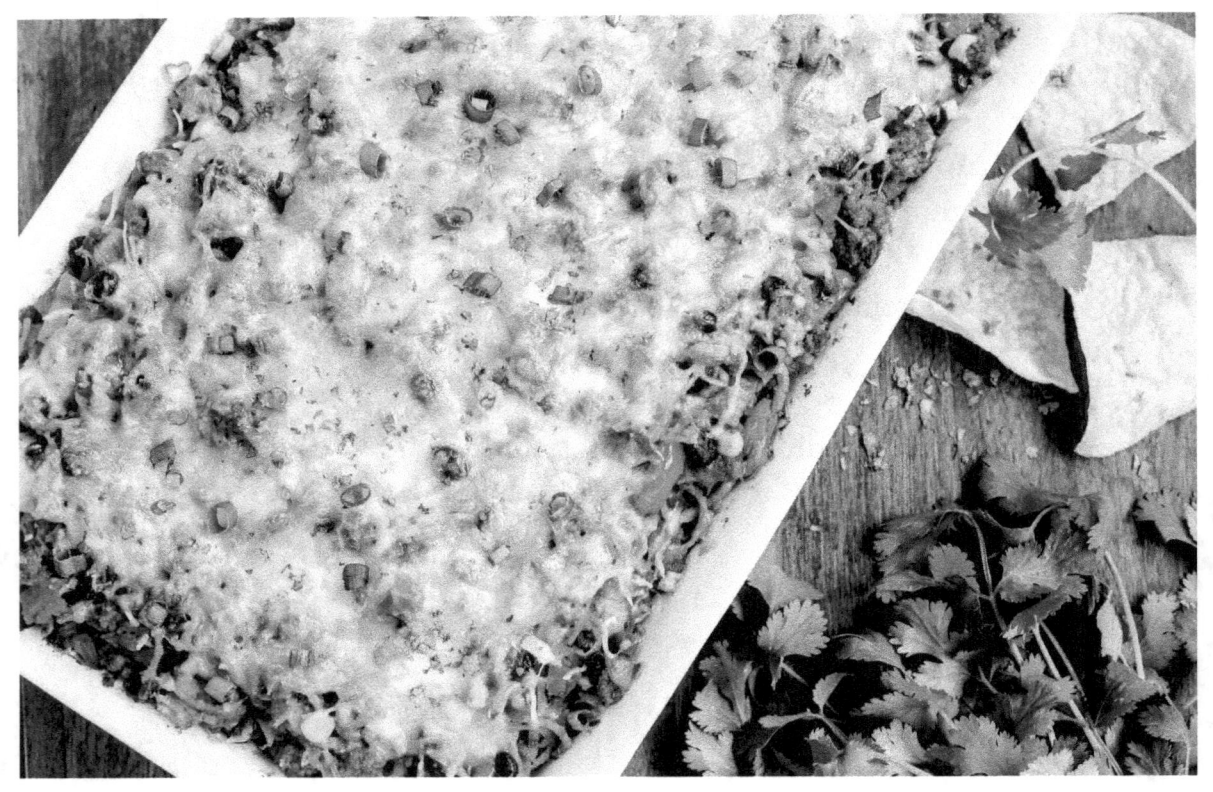

(**Freezer:** 2 months / **Microwave:** 3 ½ minutes)

8. Cabbage Fra Diavolo with beef

(**Serves:** 8 / **Prep time:** 15 minutes / **Cooking time:** 15 minutes)

Nutritional Information (Per Serving)
- 19 Grams Protein
- 28 Grams Fat
- 365 Calories
- 11 Grams Carbohydrates
- 5 Grams Fiber
- 349 milligrams sodium

Ingredients
- Ground beef (3 cups)
- Cabbage (green, 1 head)
- pepper to taste
- Butter (1 stick, unsalted)
- Pasta sauce (3 cups)
- Water (.5 cups)

Instructions
1. Take apart the cabbage and throw away the outer layers.
2. Slice into quarters and place in the food processor to shred. (If you don't want to do this, then buy cabbage that has already been shredded).
3. Put the butter in a pot and melt it down before adding the water and cabbage in along with the pepper and salt.
4. Cook for around twelve minutes, make sure to stir as to avoid burning.
5. Brown the beef while the cabbage is cooking and drain away all liquids.
6. Place beef in the cabbage pot and mix together.
7. Add pasta sauce in and mix once more.
8. Top with cheese if you want.

(**Freezer:** 1 month / **Microwave:** 3 minutes)

9. Almond bun personal pizzas

(Serves: 3 / **Prep time:** 10 minutes / **Cooking time:** 25 minutes)

Nutritional Information (Per Serving)
- 27 Grams Protein
- 653 Calories
- 4 Grams Fiber
- 56 Grams Fat
- 10 Grams Carbohydrates
- 163.3 milligrams sodium

Ingredients
- Cheddar cheese (0.0625 cups)
- Almond buns (2)
- Ground beef (1 cup)
- Pizza sauce (4 tablespoons)
- Parmesan cheese (0.0625 cups)
- Mozzarella cheese (0.125 cups)

Instructions
1. Make the almond buns (recipe can be found online).
2. Once done, put so that the flat side is facing up. This is the top of your pizza.
3. Evenly place the pizza sauce over the bun.
4. Add your toppings.
5. Add a layer of cheese.
6. Add more toppings if desired.
7. The cheese needs to be melted, and this will take about five minutes, and toppings are crisp.

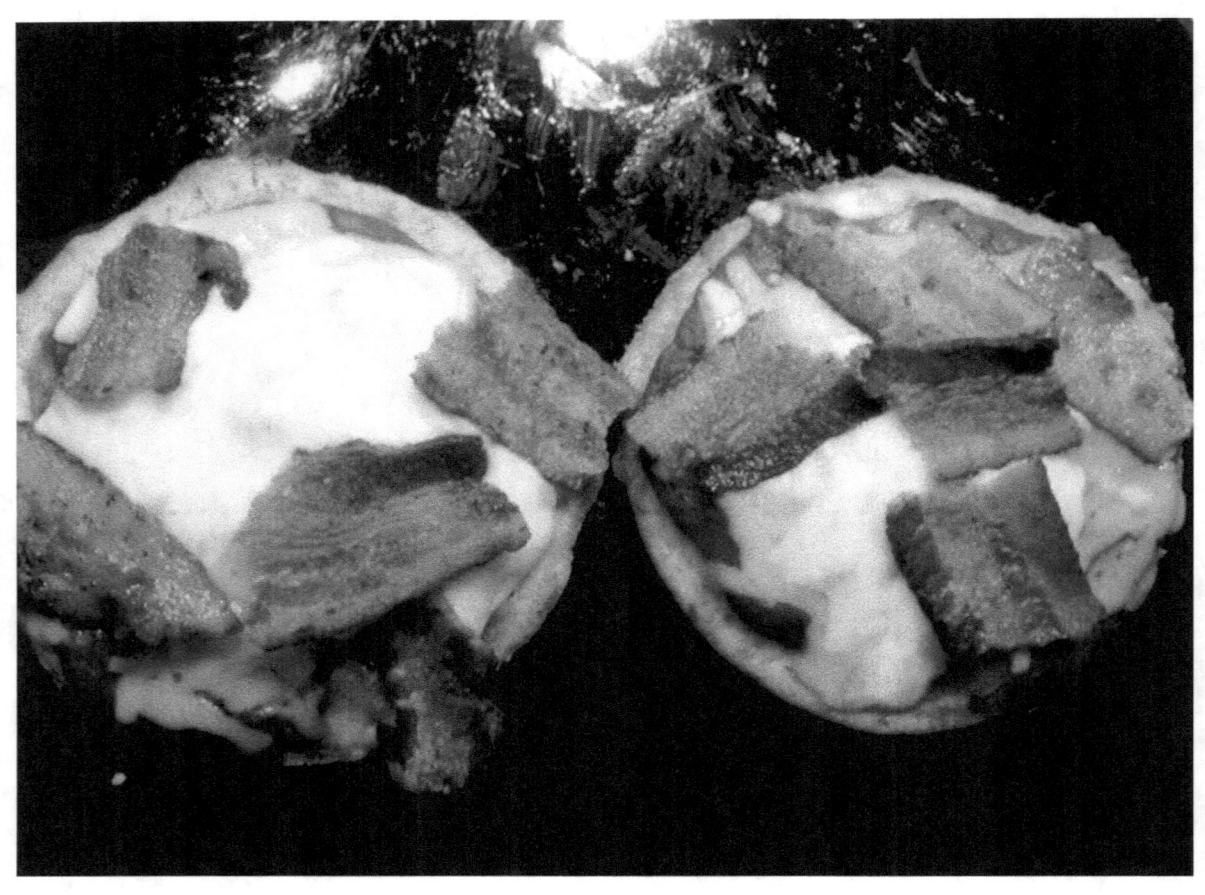

(**Freezer:** none / **Microwave:** none)

10. Bacon cheeseburger casserole

(**Serves:** 12 / **Prep time:** 20 minutes / **Cooking time:** 25 minutes)

Nutritional Information (Per Serving)
- 548 Calories
- 48.5 Grams of Protein
- 365.6 Grams Total Fat
- 4.4 Grams Carbohydrates
- 262 Milligrams Cholesterol
- 1255 Milligrams Sodium

Ingredients
- Cheddar cheese (grated, 1.5 cups)
- Ground beef (32 ounces)
- Pepper (grounded, .25 teaspoon)
- Garlic (2 cloves)
- Onion powder (.5 teaspoon)
- Heavy cream (8 ounces)
- Bacon (cooked and chopped, (16 ounces)
- Tomato paste (.75 cups)
- Eggs (8)

Instructions
1. Cook the meat with the garlic and onion until it is browned.
2. Remove grease and place on the bottom of a pan.
3. Mix in pieces of bacon.
4. Whisk eggs, heavy cream, pepper, and tomato paste together.
5. Mix in cheese to the mixture.
6. Cover meat with the mix.
7. Top off with cheese.

8. Cook for thirty-five minutes at 176.6C (350 F).

    (**Freezer:** 1 ½ months / **Microwave:** 3 minutes)

11. Kitchen sink casserole

(Serves: 12 / **Prep time:** 35 minutes / **Cooking time:** 40 minutes)

Nutritional Information (Per Serving)
- 52 Grams Protein
- 5 Carbohydrates
- 598 Calories
- 40 Grams Fat
- 1 Gram Fiber
- 1451 milligrams sodium

Ingredients
- Paprika (optional, to taste)
- Ground beef (9 cups)
- Cream cheese (2 cups)
- Onion (small, 1)
- Cheddar cheese (shredded, 1 cup)
- Celery (4 stalks)
- Bacon (7 slices)
- Sausage (3 cups)
- Cauliflower (froze, 2 cups)
- Mushrooms (sliced, 2 cups)

Instructions
1. At 204.4 C (400 F) cook the bacon in the oven for about twenty minutes.
2. Prep the rest of the meal during this time.
3. Make sure the ground beef is broken up.
4. Cook in a pan until no pink is found.
5. Brown sausage.
6. Place in a bowl without the grease.

7. Cut up the onion and celery.
8. Place in the grease and cook until translucent.
9. Unfreeze the cauliflower by cooking and then slice up.
10. Add to a large bowl.
11. Add meat to bowl after draining liquid.
12. Add bacon once done.
13. Mix in cream cheese.
14. Add cheese before mixing again.
15. Place in pan and sprinkle with paprika if you want.
16. Cook for thirty minutes at 176.6 C (350 F) be sure it is covered.
17. Uncover and cook for another 10 minutes.

(**Freezer:** 4 months / **Microwave:** 4 ½ minutes)

12. Thai pork salad with kelp noodles

(**Serves:** 2 / **Prep time:** 10 minutes / **Cooking time:** 10 minutes)

Nutritional Information (Per Serving)
Calories: 45
Carbohydrates: 14.5 g
Protein: 41
Fat: 55.3g
Fiber: 5.2 g
Sodium: 86 mg

Ingredients

- Lettuce cups (to serve with your meal)
- Your Keto approved fat of choice (1 tablespoon)
- Kelp noodles (12 ounces, you should rinse them based on what the directions on the package say)
- Ground pork (1 pound)
- White pepper (1/2 teaspoon)
- Mixed herbs (1.2 ounces, minced, cilantro, Thai basil, mint)
- Red pepper flakes (1 teaspoon)
- Ginger (2 inches, fresh, minced)
- Lime juice (3 tablespoons, fresh)
- Garlic cloves (3, minced)
- Lime zest (1 teaspoon, fresh)
- Shallots (2, sliced)
- Coconut aminos (1 tablespoon)
- Green onion (4, sliced)
- Fish sauce (1 tablespoon)

Instructions

1. Put a large skillet on the stove and heat up the fat your pork and shallots into the pan and allow them to cook for about six minutes. The pig needs to be broken up with a spoon as it cooks. After it has thoroughly browned, you are going to take a bowl and add in your garlic, half of your mixed herbs, the ginger, and green onion into a dish along with the aminos, lime zest and juice, red pepper flakes, white pepper, and fish sauce.
2. Mix your other half of the herb mix in with the pork so that the spices mix into the meat. Then add your sauce in and stir it together so that it combines all of the flavors. Place your pork in your lettuce cups and put your kelp noodles on the plate beside them.

(**Freeze:** 2 months / **Microwave**: 2 minutes)

Salads and Vegetables

1. Roquefort Pear Salad

(**Serves:** 6 / **Prep time:** 20 minutes / **Cooking time:** 10 minutes)

Nutritional Information (Per Serving)
Calories: 426
Fat: 31.6 g
Sodium: 654 mg
Carbohydrate: 33.1 g
Protein: 8 g
Fiber: 7.4 g

Ingredients
- Lettuce (1 head, torn up)
- Black pepper (to taste)
- Pears (3, peeled, cored, chopped)
- Garlic (1, chopped)
- Roquefort cheese (5 oz., crumbled)
- Mustard (1 ½ tsp)
- Avocado (1, peeled, diced, pitted)
- Sugar (1 ½ tsp)
- Onion (1/2, sliced)
- Red wine vinegar (3 tbsp.)
- Sugar (1/4 c)
- Olive oil (1/3 c)
- Pecans (1/2 c)

Instructions

1. Take a skillet and mix the ¼ cup of sugar with the pecans.
2. Stir until the sugar melts and caramelizes the pecans
3. Move the nuts to wax paper. Once cooled, break into pieces.
4. Mix the olive oil, rest of the sugar, vinegar, mustard, pepper, and garlic together
5. In a bowl, create layers of lettuce, blue cheese, avocado, onion, and pears.
6. Pour dressing over the salad
7. Sprinkle with pecan pieces

(**Freezer:** none / **Microwave:** none)

2. Mexican chopped salad

(Serves: 2 / **Prep time:** 5 minutes / **Cooking time**: none)

Nutritional Information (Per Serving)
Calories: 144
Fat: 10.4 g
Sodium: 28.8 mg
Carbohydrate: 13.8 g
Fiber: 5.0 g
Protein: 2.4 g

Ingredients
- Chili powder (3/4 tsp)
- Romaine lettuce (3 c, shredded)
- Olive oil (1/2 c)
- Red cabbage (2 c, shredded)
- Honey (1 tbsp)
- Tomato (1 c, diced)
- Jicama (1 c)
- Apple cider vinegar (3 tbsp)
- Onion (1/2 c, diced)
- Orange juice (3 tbsp)
- Cucumber (2 c, diced)
- Sunflower seeds (1/2 c, toasted)
- Avocado (1, cubed)
- Cilantro (1/2 c, chopped)

Instructions
1. Shred your lettuce and cabbage.
2. Put into a bowl.

3. Dice your other vegetables.
4. Mix your dressing ingredients together (if you make it yourself).
5. Drizzle in dressing.
6. Serve with sunflower seeds on top.

(**Freeze:** 2 months / **Microwave:** none)

3. Butternut squash and spinach salad

(**Serves:** 2 / **Prep time:** 10 minutes / **Cooking time:** 30 minutes)

Nutritional Information (Per Serving)
Calories: 198
Fiber: 5.2 g
Sodium: 19 mg
Protein: 3 g
Carbohydrates: 29.5 g

Ingredients
- Balsamic vinegar (1 c)
- Butternut squash (1, chopped)
- Raisins (1 tbsp)
- Coconut oil (3 tbsp)
- Cranberries (2 tbsp, dried)
- Shallots (2 tbsp, chopped)
- Black pepper (1/4 tsp)
- Spinach (5 oz.)

Instructions
1. Mix the squash, oil, salt, and pepper together in a bowl.
2. Spread out over a cookie sheet.
3. Cook for thirty minutes at 375 F or until the squash is turning brown.
4. Put the spinach in a bowl.
5. Dump in the shallots, cranberries, raisins, and squash.
6. Drizzle with vinegar.

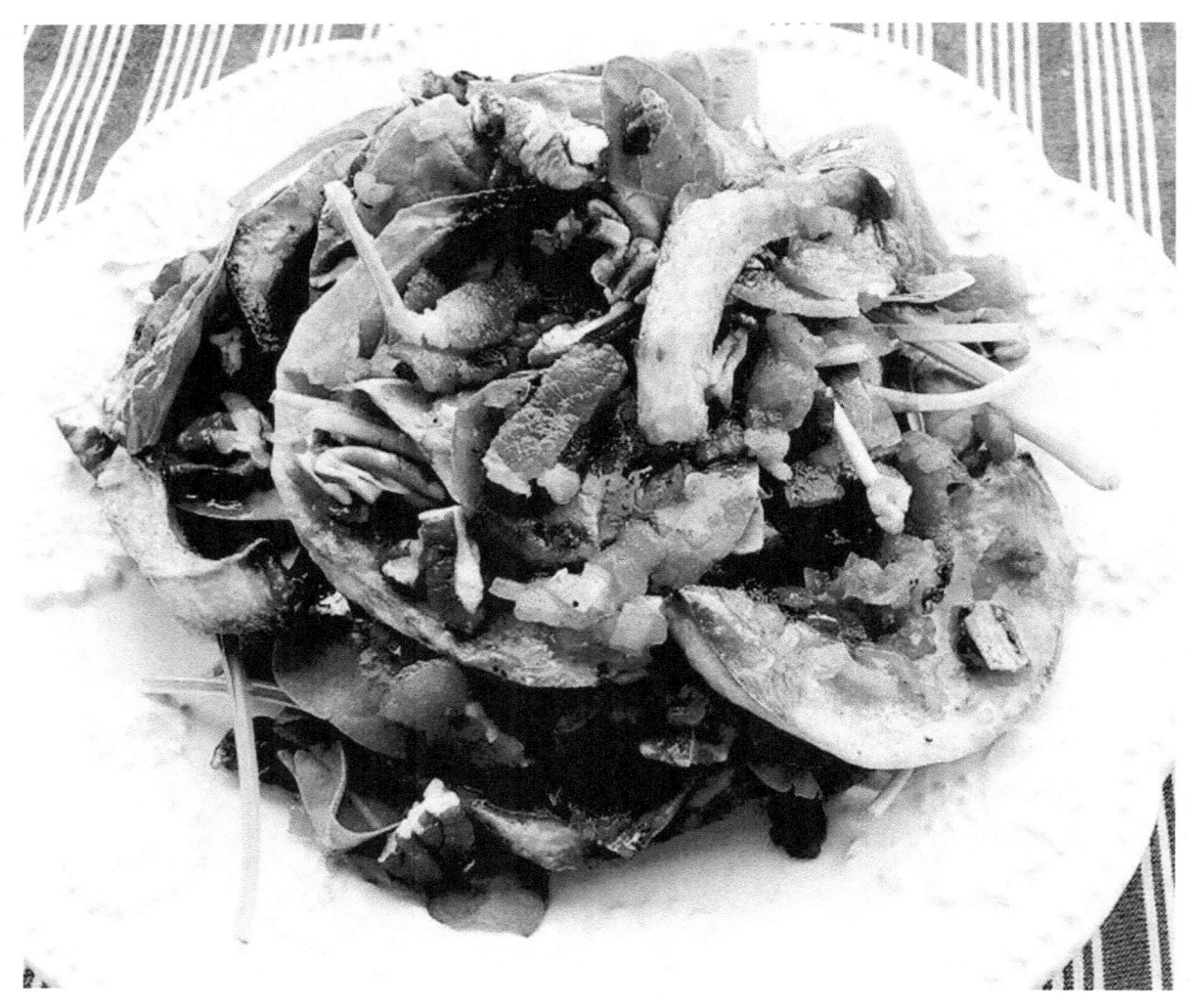

(**Freezer:** 3 months / **Microwave:** 2 minutes)

4. Fruit salad

(**Serve:** 2 / **Prep time:** 2 minutes / **Cooking time**: none)

Nutritional Information (Per Serving)
Calories: 142
Fat: 0.6 g
Carbohydrates: 34.7 g
Sodium: 12 mg
Protein: 1.8 g
Fiber: 3.4 g

Ingredients
- Honey (1 tbsp, raw)
- Orange (1)
- Coconut (1/2 c, shredded)
- Blueberries (1/2 c)
- Cinnamon (1/2 tsp)
- Blackberries (1/2 c)
- Strawberries (8)
- Grapes (1/2 c)
- Kiwi (2, sliced)

Instructions
1. Mix all of your fruits together in a bowl.
2. Drizzle with honey.
3. Put cinnamon on top.

(**Freezer:** none / **Microwave:** none)

5. Skirt steak avocado salad

(**Serves:** 2 / **Prep time:** 10 minutes / **Cooking time:** 10 minutes)

Nutritional Information (Per Serving)
Calories: 310
Fat: 19 g
Sodium: 574 mg
Carbohydrate: 12 g
Fiber: 5.3 g

Ingredients
- Lime juice (2 tsp)
- Skirt steak (2 lb.)
- Cilantro (2 tsp, chopped) coconut oil (4 tbsp)
- Chili powder (1/2 tsp)
- Onion (1, diced)
- Paprika (1/2 tsp)
- Poblano pepper (1)
- Cumin (1/2 tsp)
- Tomatoes (2, diced)
- Avocado (1, pitted, cubed)

Instructions
1. Put your grill on a medium heat.
2. Cut up the tomatoes, avocado, onion, and pepper tossing it into a bowl.
3. Chop the cilantro and lime before putting in a separate bowl and putting in the fridge.
4. In another bowl, mix the oil, chili powder, paprika, and cumin.
5. Cover your steak in your seasoning mixture.
6. Grill for five minutes a side.

7. Remove and allow to cool.
8. Slice into strips.
9. Mix with your salad and enjoy.

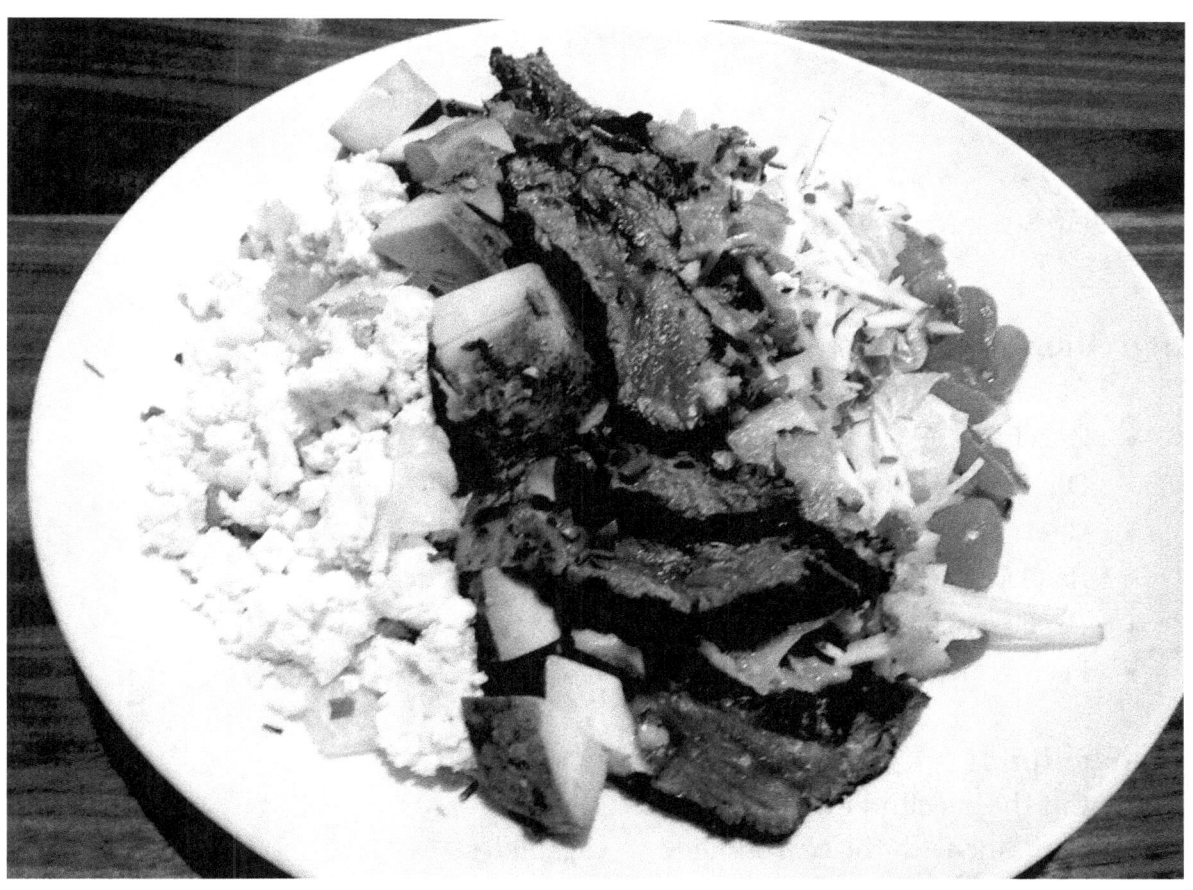

(**Freezer:** 6 months / **Microwave:** 4 minutes)

6. Zucchini pasta salad

(**Serves:** 2 / **Prep time:** 5 minutes / **Cooking time:** none)

Nutritional Information (Per Serving)

Calories: 147

Fat: 11.1 g

Sodium: 391 mg

Carbohydrates: 9.1 g

Protein: 5 g

Fiber: 2.1 g

Ingredients

- Balsamic vinegar (1 tbsp)
- Zucchini (1)
- Olive oil (2 tbsp)
- Cherry tomatoes (8)
- Basil (2 tbsp, fresh)
- Garlic cloves (1, minced)
- Pecans (1/4 c)

Instructions

1. Cut the zucchini into long strips.
2. Combine with the seasonings and vegetables.
3. Toss together.

(**Freezer:** 4 months / **Microwave:** 3 minutes)

7. Cranberry spinach salad

(**Serves:** 2 / **Prep time:** 10 minutes / **Cooking time:** 10 minutes)

Nutritional Information (Per Serving)
Calories: 338
Fat: 23.5 g
Fiber: 3.6 g
Sodium: 58 mg
Carbohydrate: 30.4 g
Protein: 4.9 g

Ingredients
- Balsamic vinegar (1 tbsp)
- Spinach (1/2 lb.)
- Olive oil (1/2 c)
- Chicken breast (1, boneless)
- Coconut oil (1 tsp)
- Cashews (1/4 c, unsalted)
- Sesame seeds (2 tsp, toasted)
- Cranberries (1 c, dried)
- Carrot (1/2 c, sliced)

Instructions
1. Heat your skillet and melt the coconut oil in it.
2. Cook your chicken in the skillet. Make sure that it is entirely done.
3. Take your carrots and slice them into strips.
4. After the chicken has cooled, you will cut it into long pieces.
5. In a bowl take the vinegar, olive oil, and sesame seeds and mix it all together.
6. Mix the spinach into the pan along with the cashews and cranberries.
7. Mix everything together and enjoy it.

(**Freezer:** none / **Microwave:** none)

8. Kale Caesar salad

(**Serves:** 4 / **Prep time:** 20 minutes / **Cooking time:** 25 minutes)

Nutritional Information (Per Serving)
Carbohydrates: 8.4 g
Protein: 10.5 g
Fat: 36.6 g
Calories: 115
Fiber: 3.5 g
Sodium: 481 mg

Ingredients
Salad

- Parmesan (1/4 c)
- Kale (1/2 lb.)
- Garlic powder (1/2 tsp)
- Olive oil (3 tbsp)
- Keto Focaccia (1 batch)

Dressing

- Parmesan (3 tbsp)
- Garlic cloves (3)
- Mayonnaise (3/4 c)
- Anchovy paste (1 tbsp)
- Dijon mustard (2 tsp)
- Worcestershire sauce (2 tsp)
- Lemon juice (2 tbsp)

Instructions
1. Preheat oven to 375F.

2. Cut the focaccia into cubes and toss in oil and garlic. Place on a sheet and cook for fifteen minutes.
3. Place dressing ingredients in a jar.
4. Shake and chill.
5. Cover kale in dressing.
6. Place focaccia on top.

(Freezer: none / **Microwave:** none)

9. Low carb rainbow salad with feta

(**Serves:** 3 / **Prep time:** 15 minutes / **Cooking time:** none)

Nutritional Information (Per Serving)
Carbohydrates: 12.7 g
Protein: 10.8 g
Fat: 37.1 g
Calories: 200
Fiber: 4 g
Sodium: 116 mg

Ingredients
- Feta (2/3 c)
- White cabbage (1 c)
- Pumpkin seeds (1/3 c)
- Radishes (3/4 c)
- Peppers (red, 3)
- Carrot (1)
- Cucumber (1/2)
- Zucchini (1/2)

Instructions
1. Peel all ingredients and cut into bite-sized pieces.
2. Toss in a bowl.
3. Cover with feta.
4. Coat in dressing of your choice.

(**Freezer:** none / **Microwave:** none)

10. Sweet and spicy pickled jalapenos

(**Serves:** 16 / **Prep time:** 10 minutes / **Cooking time:** 20 minutes)

Nutritional Information (Per Serving)
Calories: 30
Carbohydrates: 1.8 g
Fat: 0.1 g
Protein: 0.2 g
Fiber: 0.5 g
Sodium: 3 mg

Ingredients
- Cayenne pepper (1/4 tsp)
- Jalapeno peppers (20)
- Onion powder (1/2 tsp)
- Water (1 ½ c)
- Garlic powder (1/2 tsp)
- Apple cider vinegar (1/4 c)
- Swerve (6 oz.)

Instructions
1. Cut up your peppers.
2. Mix with the rest of the ingredients in a bowl.
3. Boil on the stove and simmer for ten minutes.
4. Place a jar and put in the fridge for 2 weeks.

(**Freezer:** none / **Microwave:** none)

11. Refrigerator pickles

(**Serves:** 1 jar / **Prep time:** 20 minutes / **Cooking time**: none)

Nutritional Information (Per Serving)
Carbohydrates: 1.5 g
Calories: 20
Protein: 0.3 g
Fiber: 0.6
Fat: 0.1 g
Sodium: 0 g

Ingredients
- Apple cider vinegar (1 c)
- Cucumbers (12)
- Water (2 c)
- Peppercorns (1 tsp)
- Swerve (4 tbsp)
- Mustard seeds (1 tsp)
- Garlic cloves (2)
- All spice (5)
- Onion (1)
- Bay leaf (1)
- Dill seeds (1 tsp)

Instructions
1. Slice the cucumbers into spears.
2. Make your pickling brine in a saucepan by heating up the water and vinegar. You are going to want to allow the swerve to melt in the liquid before adding the garlic and onion.
3. Place the spices in a jar.
4. Insert pickles and cover in juice.
5. Place in fridge for 3 months.

(**Freezer:** none / **Microwave:** none)

12. Lemon roasted broccoli

(Serves: 4 / **Prep time:** 5 minutes / **Cooking time:** 15 minutes)

Nutritional Information (Per Serving)
Fat: 14.3 g
Carbohydrates: 10.9 g
Protein: 4.3 g
Calories: 124.2
Fiber: 2.7 g
Sodium: 326 mg

Ingredients
- Broccoli (1.3 lb.)
- Lemon juice (2 tbsp)
- Ghee (1/4 c)
- Garlic cloves (2)

Instructions
1. Preheat oven to 450 F and cut broccoli into florets.
2. Mix with garlic and ghee.
3. Cook for 15 minutes.

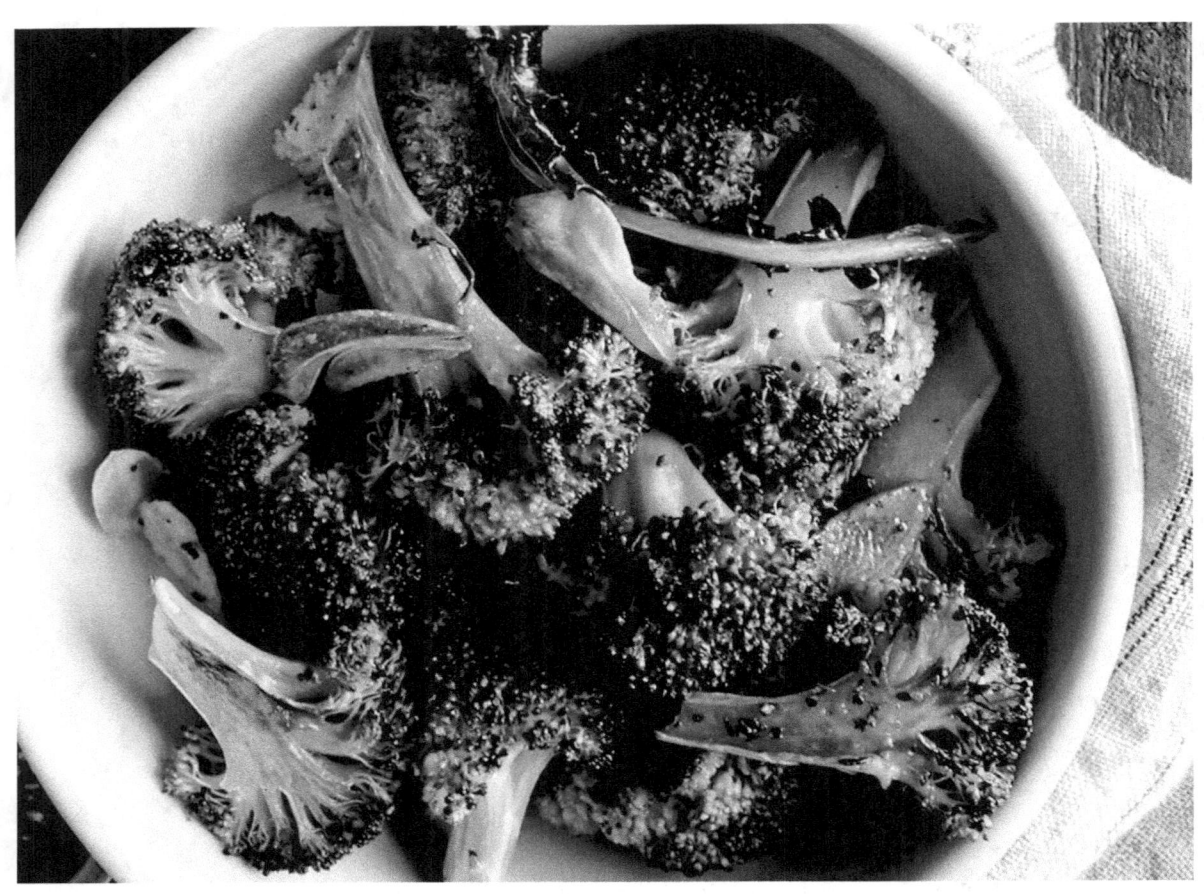

(**Freezer:** 2 months / **Microwave:** 2 minutes)

13. Garlic red potatoes

(**Serves:** 4 / **Prep time:** 10 minutes / **Cooking time:** 40 minutes)

Nutritional Information (Per Serving)
Calories: 279
Fat: 7.6 g
Protein: 5.3 g
Carbohydrates: 39.6 g
Fiber: 9.9 g
Sodium: 77 mg

Ingredients
1. Parmesan cheese (1 tablespoon)
2. Red potatoes (2 pounds)
3. Lemon (1, juiced)
4. Butter (1/4 cup, melted)
5. Salt (1 teaspoon)
6. Garlic (2 teaspoons, minced)

Instructions
1. Turn the oven on to 350 F
2. Once you have cut the potatoes up and place them in an 8x8 dish
3. Mix the spices with the butter and lemon juice before dumping over the potatoes and stirring to ensure they are coated properly.
4. Sprinkle cheese over the potatoes
5. Bake covered for 30 minutes. Uncover and continue to bake for 10 more minutes.

(**Freezer:** 1 month / **Microwave:** 1 ½ minutes)

Snacks and Sides

1. Cheese and chive scones

(**Serves:** 15 / **Prep time:** 15 minutes / **Cooking time:** 25 minutes)

Nutritional Information (Per Serving)
Carbohydrates: 3.5 g
Protein: 5.7 g
Fat: 10.4 g
Calories: 115
Sodium: 193.3 mg
Fiber: 0.9 g

Ingredients
- Black pepper (1/2 tsp)
- Almond flour (1 ½ c)
- Eggs (2)
- Coconut flour (1/4 c)
- Almond milk (3 tbsp)
- Flax seeds (1/4 c)
- Cheddar cheese (1.8 oz.)
- Baking powder (1 tsp)
- Chives (2)
- Bacon (4 slices)

Instructions
1. Turn the oven on to 375 F.
2. Blitz the flax seeds in your blender.
3. Mix the flours, seeds, baking powder, cheese, chives, and pepper in a bowl.

4. Cut up the bacon and fry it.
5. Crack the eggs and mix with the almond milk.
6. Add in the dry ingredients to the wet ones.
7. Roll out onto grease paper.
8. Cut into scones.
9. Bake for 15 minutes.

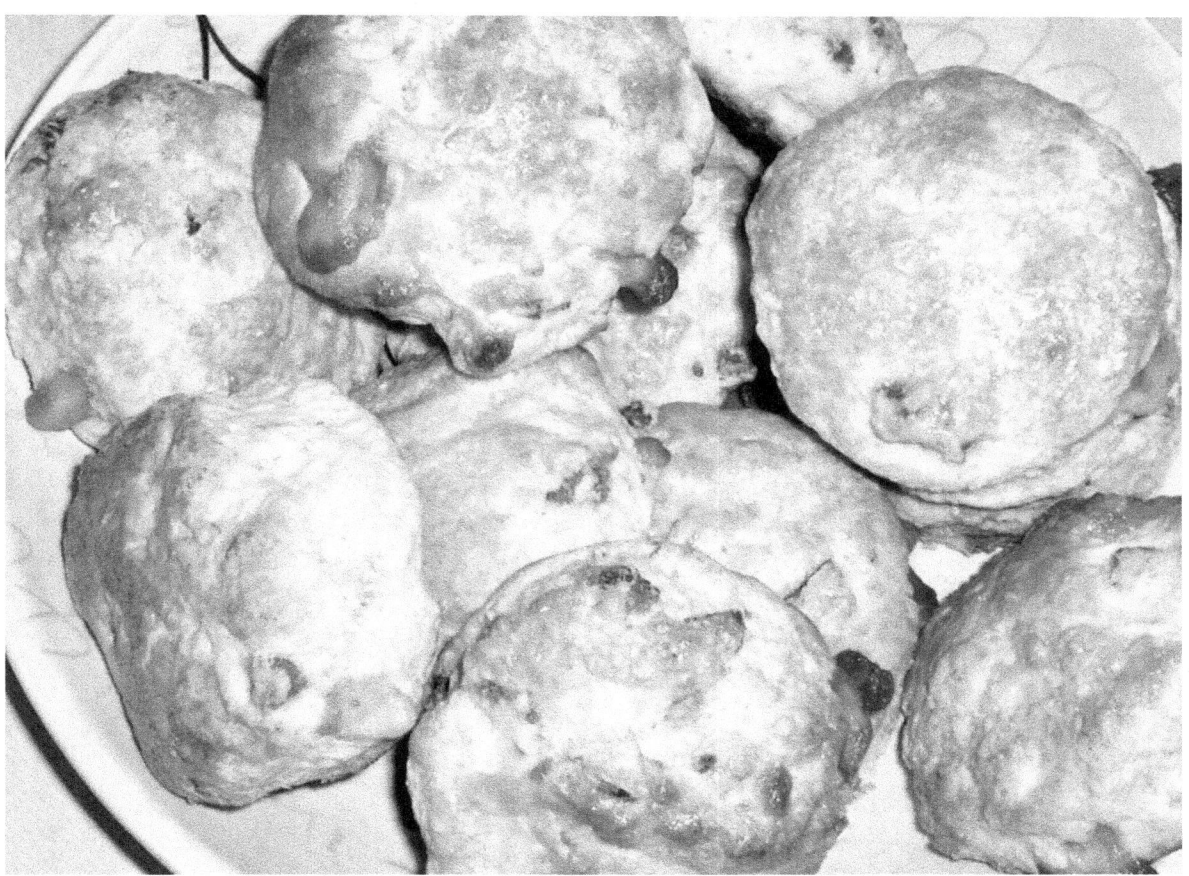

(**Freezer:** none / **Microwave:** none)

2. Kale Slaw

(**Serves:** 6 / **Prep time:** 10 minutes / **Cooking time:** 10 minutes)

Nutritional Information (Per Serving)
Protein: 3.4 g
Carbohydrates: 6 g
Fat: 13.3 g
Calories: 147
Sodium: 245 mg
Fiber: 3 g

Ingredients
- Kale (6 oz.)
- Lemon juice (1 tbsp)
- Red cabbage (2 ½ c)
- Mayonnaise (1/3 c)
- Green cabbage (1 ¼ c)
- Pumpkin seeds (1/4 c)
- Carrot (1/2 c)

Instructions
1. Slice the kale into a bowl.
2. Slice the cabbages into the same pot.
3. Add in the carrot.
4. Dress in mayo and lemon juice.

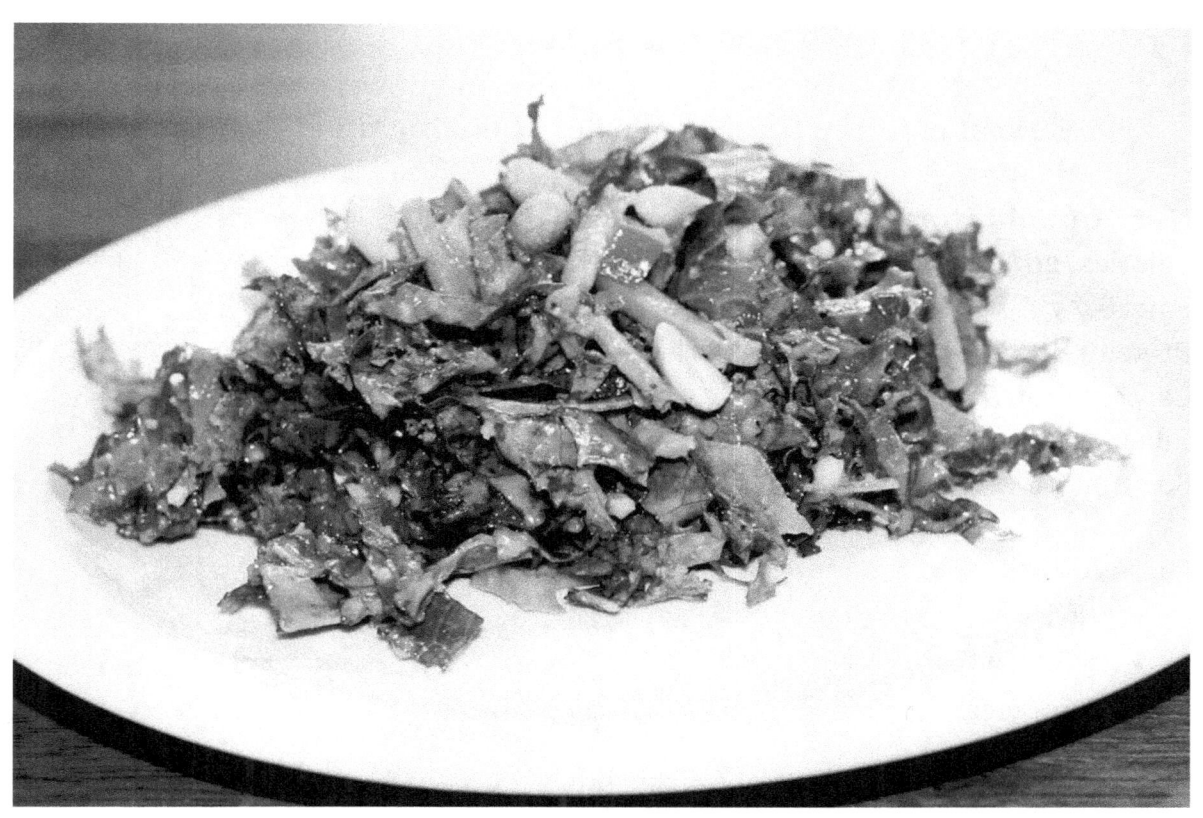

(**Freezer:** none / **Microwave:** none)

3. Cheesy bacon dip

(**Serves:** 12 / **Prep time:** 15 minutes / **Cooking time:** 45 minutes)

Nutritional Information (Per Serving)
Calories: 201
Fat: 18.7 g
Protein: 8.3 g
Carbohydrates: 2.8 g
Fiber: 0.2 g
Sodium: 219.2 mg

Ingredients
- Swiss cheese (2 c)
- Ghee (2 tbsp)
- Sour cream (1 c)
- Onion (1)
- Cream cheese (1 c)
- Chili pepper (1)
- Bacon (8 slices)

Instructions
1. Preheat oven to 350 F.
2. Cook ghee, onion, and pepper for ten minutes.
3. Add in the bacon.
4. In a bowl mix the cream cheese and sour cream.
5. Grate in cheese and mix well.
6. Remove grease and place in the bowl with the cheese but do not put the bacon grease in the pan.
7. Spread evenly in a container and cook for 35 minutes.

(**Freezer:** 2 months / **Microwave:** 3 ½ minutes)

4. Meatballs

(**Serves:** 25 / **Prep time:** 15 minutes / **Cooking time:** 30 minutes)

Nutritional Information (Per Serving)
Calories: 117
Carbohydrates: 1.4 g
Protein: 7 g
Fat: 9.3 g
Fiber: 0.3 g
Sodium: 333 mg

Ingredients
- Pepper (to taste)
- Ground beef (1.1 g)
- Mozzarella (1 c)
- Egg (1)
- Almond flour (1/2 c)
- Garlic clove (2)
- Thyme (1 tsp)
- Oregano (1 tsp)

Instructions
1. Heat oven to 450 F.
2. Dice up cheese and put in the freezer.
3. Put meat, garlic, thyme, oregano, and egg in bowl with almond flour
4. Mix well.
5. Divide out.
6. Put cheese in the middle of each meatball.
7. Cook for fifteen minutes.

(**Freezer:** 4 months / **Microwave:** 2 ½ minutes)

5. Easy Guacamole

(**Serves:** 4 / **Prep time:** 10 minutes / **Cooking time**: none)

Nutritional Information (Per Serving)
Calories: 181
Protein: 2.8 g
Fat: 14.9 g
Carbohydrates: 13.2 g
Fiber: 2 g
Sodium: 2 mg

Ingredients
- Avocados (2)
- Black pepper (to taste)
- Cherry tomatoes (1 1/3 c)
- Cilantro (4 tbsp)
- Onion (1)
- Red chili pepper (1)
- Garlic cloves (2)
- Lime juice (4 tbsp)

Instructions
1. Peel the onion and chop the pepper and tomato.
2. Peel and halve avocados. Mash with a fork.
3. Place lime juice, onion, garlic, and tomatoes, and pepper into the avocado.
4. Mix together.

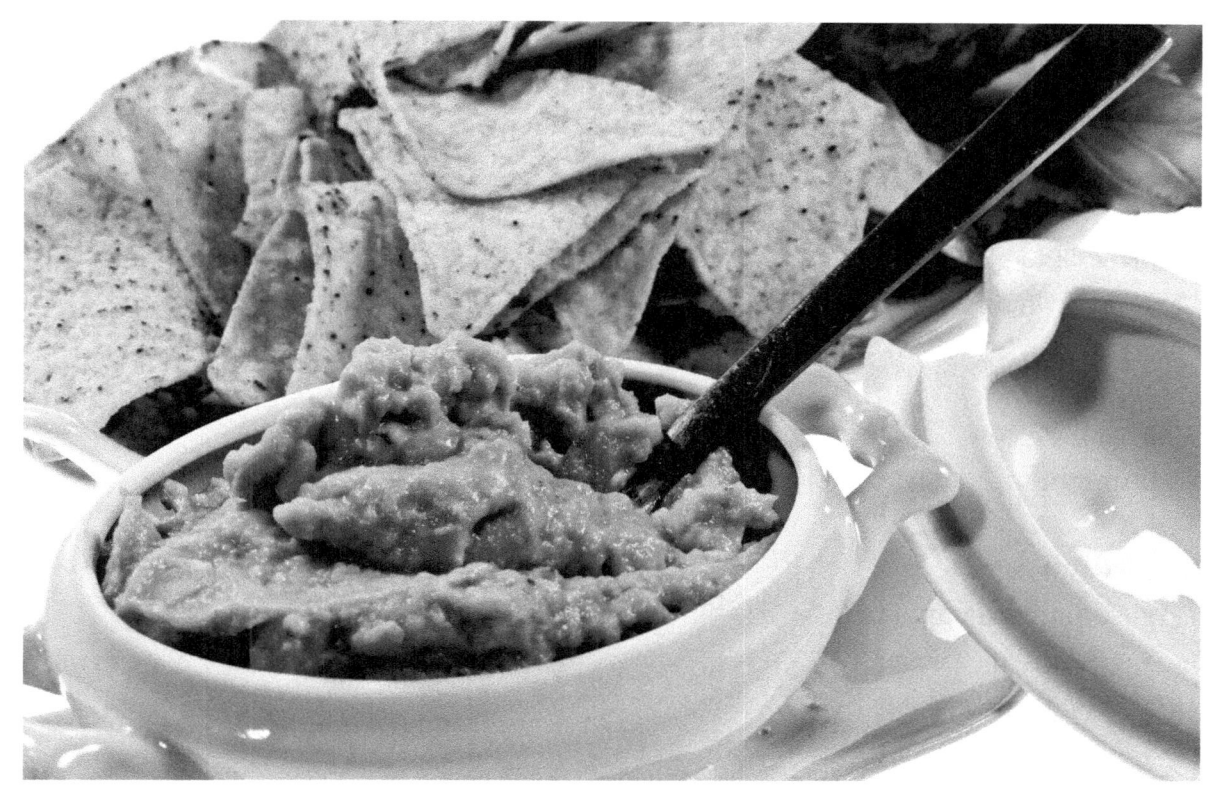

(**Freezer:** 4 months / **Microwave:** none)

6. Bacon and gruyere jalapeno poppers

(**Serves:** 4 / **Prep time:** 10 minutes / **Cooking time:** 35 minutes)

Nutritional Information (Per Serving)
Calories: 434
Carbohydrates: 4.7 g
Fat: 35.5 g
Protein: 24.2 g
Fiber: 1.2 g
Sodium: 32 mg

Ingredients
- Jalapeno peppers (12)
- Cilantro (2 tbsp)
- Ricotta cheese (1 c)
- Bacon (12)
- Gruyere (1/2 c)

Instructions
1. Preheat over 400 F
2. Deseed and half the peppers
3. Mix ricotta, gruyere, and cilantro
4. Fill each pepper
5. Wrap in bacon
6. Cook for 25 minutes

(**Freezer:** 5 months / **Microwave:** none)

7. Rosemary garlic eggplant chips

(**Serves:** 4 / **Prep time:** 10 minutes / **Cooking time:** 40 minutes)

Nutritional Information (Per Serving)
Calories: 133
Carbohydrates: 7.5 g
Protein: 1.3 g
Fat: 11.5
Fiber: 4.3 g
Sodium: 296 mg

Ingredients
- Rosemary (1 tbsp)
- Eggplants (2)
- Garlic cloves (1)
- Ghee (3 tbsp)

Instructions
1. Slice eggplant into ½ cm pieces.
2. Put on cookie sheet and season. Allow for leaching before placing in the oven.
3. Heat oven to 350 F.
4. Coat in oil mix.
5. Cook for 30 minutes.

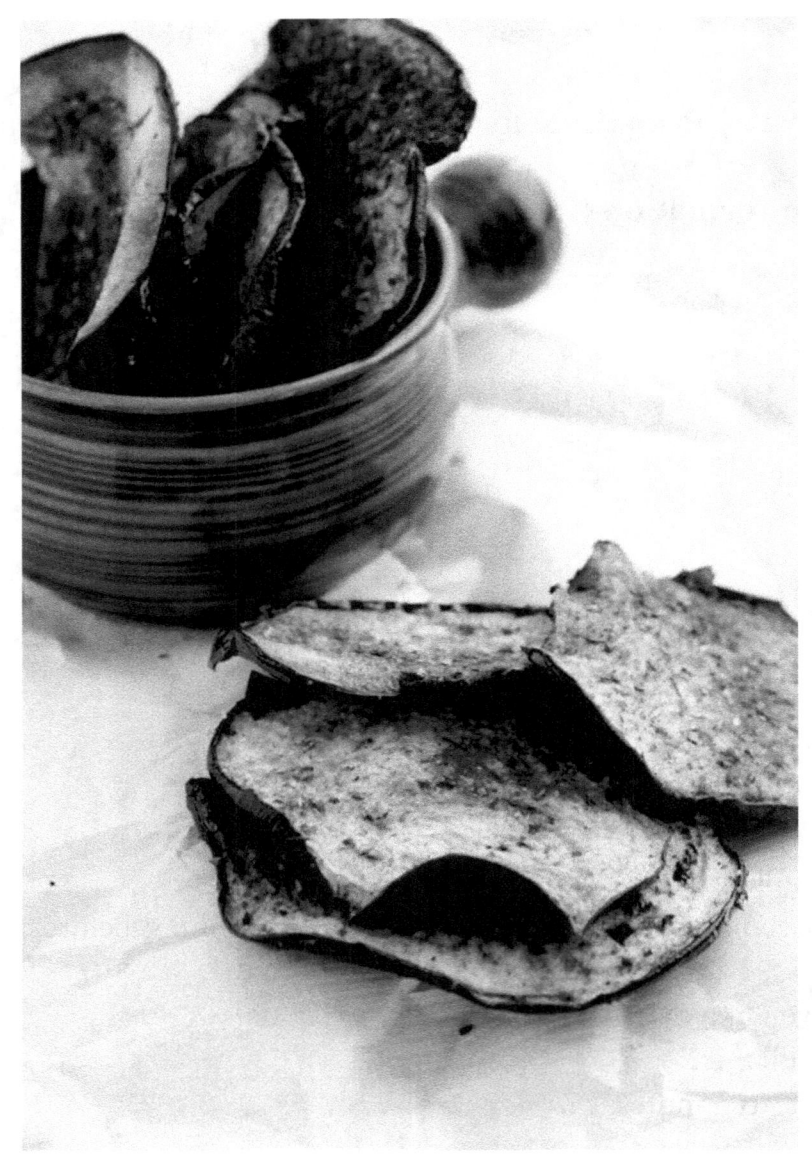

(**Freezer:** 8 months / **Microwave:** 1 ½ minutes)

8. Mushroom Chips

(**Serves:** 4 / **Prep time:** 15 minutes / **Cooking time:** 1 hour)

Nutritional Information (Per Serving)
Calories: 169
Carbohydrates: 5.8 g
Protein: 3.2 g
Fat: 15.5 g
Fiber: 0.6 g
Sodium: 2.8 mg

Ingredients
- Black pepper (to taste)
- Portobello mushrooms (10.6 oz.)
- Ghee (4 tbsp)

Instructions
1. Turn on the oven to 300 F.
2. Slice mushrooms thinly.
3. Put on a cookie sheet and coat in oil.
4. Cook for 60 minutes.

(**Freezer:** 3 months / **Microwave:** none)

9. Mocha lace biscuits

(**Serves:** 18 / **Prep time:** 10 minutes / **Cooking time:** 30 minutes)

Nutritional Information (Per Serving)
Calories: 95
Protein: 1.9 g
Carbohydrates: 6
Fat: 8.5 g
Fiber: 4.4 g
Sodium: 28 mg

Ingredients
- Instant coffee powder (2 tsp)
- Ghee (1/2 c)
- Shredded coconut (0.7 oz.)
- swerve (1/4 c)
- cacao powder (1/2c)
- maple syrup (4 tbsp)
- almond meal (1 c)
- vanilla extract (1 tsp)

Instructions
1. Preheat oven to 375 F.
2. Put ghee, swerve, syrup and vanilla in a pan and allow to melt.
3. Place dry ingredients into bowl and mix.
4. Pour into wet ingredients and mix well.
5. Use a spoon and set on a baking tray.
6. Cook for 12 minutes.

(**Freezer:** 1 year / **Microwave:** none)

10. Raspberry chia pudding

(Serves: 4 / **Prep time:** 5 minutes / **Cooking time:** none)

Nutritional Information (Per Serving)
Calories: 183
Fat: 9.2 g
Carbohydrates: 12.9 g
Protein: 5.5 g
Fiber: 12.7 g
Sodium: 33 mg

Ingredients
- Unsweetened almond milk or plant milk of your choice (1 cup)
- Vanilla powder (1 teaspoon)
- Water (1/2 cup)
- Chia seeds (1/2 cup, whole)
- Raspberries (1 cup, fresh or frozen, choice is yours)

Instructions
1. In a blender, blend the raspberries, milk, and water. Don't use all of the raspberries because you will want some for a topping on your pudding.
2. The chia seeds will need to be mixed with the blended mixture as well as the vanilla. You can add the sweetener if you are using it.
3. For twenty-five minutes, allow the mixture to sit.
4. Serve topped with the rest of your raspberries.

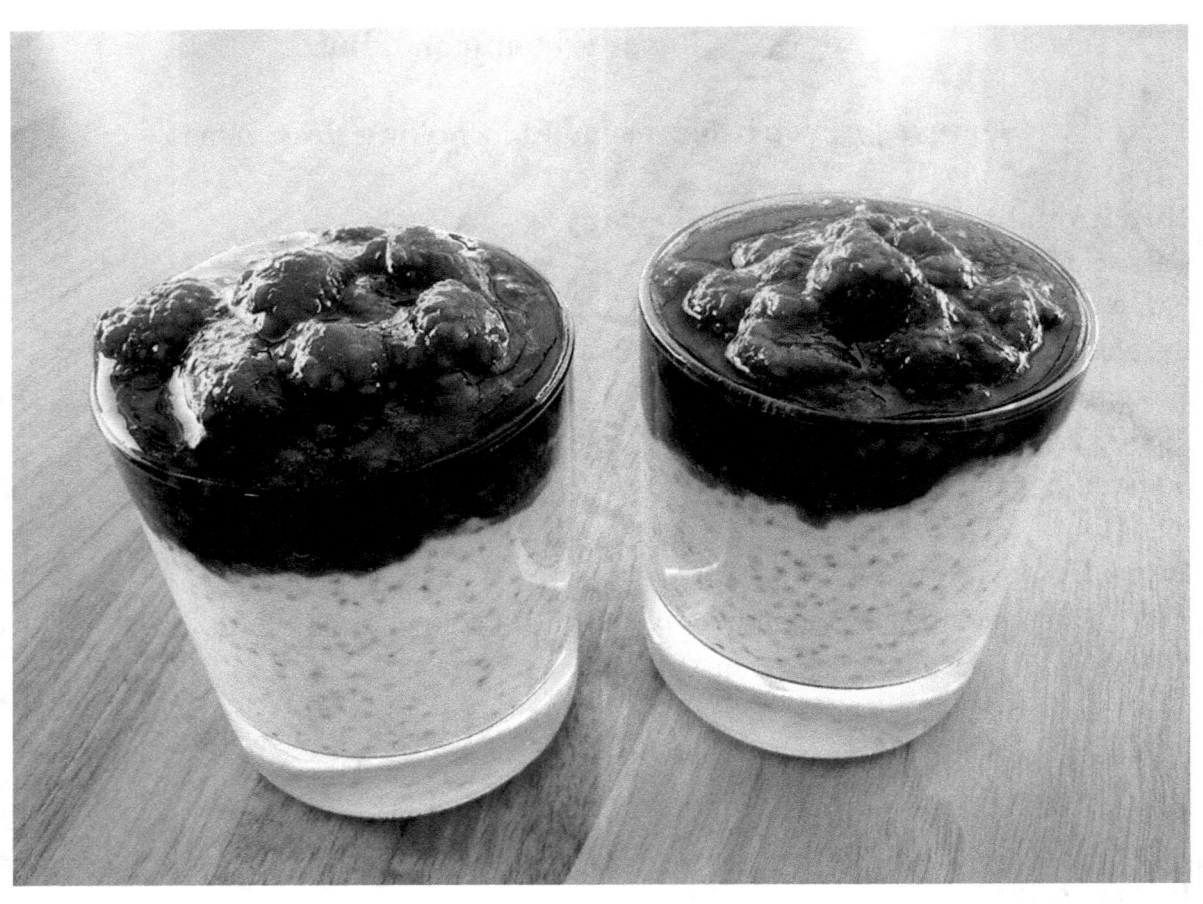

(**Freezer:** 1 year / **Microwave:** none)

11. Almond flour coconut oil brownies

(**Serves:** 15 / **Prep time:** 15 minutes / **Cooking time:** 15 minutes)

Nutritional Information (Per Serving)
Calories: 169
Carbohydrates: 7.3
Fat: 14.8 g
Protein: 5.1
Fiber: 2.9 g
Sodium: 18 mg

Ingredients
- Stevia (15 drops)
- Almond flour (1 cup)
- Baking soda (1/2 teaspoon)
- Dark chocolate (3/4 cup)
- Himalayan salt (½ teaspoon)
- Dates (1/2 cup, seedless)
- Coconut oil (1/2 cup, melted)
- Eggs (3)

Instructions
1. With your food processor, you'll pulse the flour, salt, and baking soda together.
2. Now, you'll pulse your dark chocolate in until you get a rough texture.
3. Lastly, put the rest of the ingredients in and continue to pulse them until everything is smooth.
4. In a baking dish, line it with baking paper before pouring your brownie mix into it.
5. Use a spatula to even your mixture out.

6. Place your brownies in the oven at 320 F for fifteen minutes. You will need to keep an eye on your brownies to ensure they do not burn.

   (**Freezer:** 6 months / **Microwave:** 2 minutes)

12. Chocolate and mint smoothie

(**Serves:** 1 / **Prep time:** 5 minutes / **Cooking time:** N/A)

Nutritional Information (Per Serving)
Calories: 401
Carbohydrates; 14.3 g
Protein: 5
Fat: 40.3 g
Fiber: 2.3 g
Sodium: 118.1 mg

Ingredients
- Ice cubes (a few)
- Almond milk (1 cup, unsweetened)
- MCT oil (1 tablespoon)
- Coconut milk (1/4 cup)
- Erythritol (2 tablespoons, powdered)
- Avocado (1/2)
- Mint (a few leaves)
- Cocoa powder (1 tablespoon)

Instructions
1. Put the ingredients in the blender.
2. Throw in a few ice cubes and mix until it is entirely smooth.
3. You can top with some whipped coconut cream.

(**Freezer:** none / **Microwave:** none)

13. Gluten-free almond flour chocolate chip cookies

(Serves: 14 / **Prep time**: 10 minutes / **Cooking time:** 10 minutes)

Nutritional Information (Per Serving)
Calories: 162
Fat: 12.4 g
Protein: 4.2 g
Carbohydrates: 10.6 g
Fiber: 2.1 g
Sodium: 108 mg

Ingredients
1. Chocolate chips (1/2 cup)
2. Brown sugar (1/4 cup)
3. Baking soda (1/2 teaspoon)
4. King Arthur almond flour (2 cups)
5. Salt (1/4 teaspoon)
6. Egg (1)
7. Butter (2 tablespoons)
8. Vanilla extract (2 teaspoons)

Instructions

1. Turned the oven on to 350 F. grease a baking sheet.
2. Mix the baking soda, salt, butter, and brown sugar until the mix is smooth
3. Combine the vanilla, almond flour and egg. Scrape the bottom and the sides of the bowl as you mix the batter for one minute.
4. Add in the chocolate chips.
5. Create small balls of dough on the cookie sheet. You may want to use a cookie scoop.
6. Flatten the cookies down to $3/8^{th}$ inch thick.

7. Cook for twelve minutes
8. Take out of the oven and them to cool for two minutes before placing them on a cooling rack.

(Freezer: none / **Microwave:** none)

Conclusion

Thank you for making it through to the end of *The Healthy Meal Prep Cookbook*, let's hope it was informative and able to provide you with all of the tools you need to achieve your goals, whatever they may be.

The next step is to start your meal prep. You will realize that meal prep will change your life and make your days go by a lot faster. Meal prep will make it to where you can stick to your low carb diet which will help you lose weight and have the lifestyle you want.

The recipes that you found in this book will be recipes that will help you lose weight and keep it off! Whenever you lose weight, you will be living a healthier life, and that will make you happier.

One of the best things to remember is to stay away from the salt! Salt retains water, and that is not something you want to take up residence in your body!

Finally, before you go, I'd like to say "thank you" for purchasing my book.
I know you could have picked from dozens of books on Meal Prep, but you took a chance with my guide. So, big thanks for downloading this book and reading all the way to the end.

Now, I'd like to ask for a *small* favor. Could you please take a minute or two and leave a review for this book on Amazon? This feedback will help me continue to write the kind of books that will help you get results.

Thank you and good luck!

Recipe Index

A

Almond bun personal pizzas 181
Almond flour coconut oil brownies 225
Apple, pear, and walnut salad 106
Asparagus with browned butter and creamy eggs 41

B

Bacon and gruyere jalapeno poppers 218
Bacon cheeseburger casserole 183
Bacon Hash 43
Barbecue Tofu sandwiches 110
Beef and egg stuffed pattypan squash 166
Beef and pumpkin breakfast casserole 59
Beef and winter vegetable soup 70
Breakfast stuffed peppers 48
Butternut squash and spinach salad 193

C

Cabbage Fra Diavolo with beef 179
Cauliflower soup with crumbled pancetta 64
Cheese and chive scones 210
Cheesy bacon dip 214
Cheesy beef casserole 177
Chia Seed Crackers and roasted red pepper and goat cheese dip 92

Chicken and vegetable soup 72
Chicken bacon crock pot chowder 86
Chicken fajitas 145
Chicken Salad Lettuce Wraps 141
Chicken soup 66
Chicken tomato and green bean curry 161
Chicken with cauliflower and olives 159
Chili lime crispy chicken wings 143
Chili soup 76
Chocolate and mint smoothie 227
Cracklin' chicken 153
Cranberry spinach salad 199
Creamy white chili 90
Czech Christmas fried fish 116

E

Easy Guacamole 216
Easy spicy crockpot double beef stew 74
Egg drop soup 99
Eggplant and lamb soup 67
Eggplant parmesan 115

F

Fish cakes with aioli 118
Fruit salad 195

G

Garlic red potatoes 209

Gluten-free almond flour chocolate chip cookies 228
Grain Free Breakfast Taco Pie Filling 168
Grandma's spaghetti soup 78
Green smoothie 51
Grilled chicken breasts with zucchini 155
Grilled fish steaks 136
Grilled lobster 121
Grilled Portobello Mushrooms with Mashed Cannellini Beans and Harissa
    Sauce 113
Grilled veggie and grilled chicken salads with tomato vinaigrette 149

I

Inside Out Scotch Eggs 45

K

Kale Caesar salad 201
Kale Slaw 212
Keto harissa chicken skewers 157
Keto Iced Coffee 54
Kitchen sink casserole 185

L

Lemon roasted broccoli 207
Low carb chicken fricassee 147
Low carb Greek briam 101
Low carb lemon poppy seed muffins 62
Low carb rainbow salad with feta 203
Low carb Starbucks pink drink 47

M

Macadamia crusted sea bass mango cream sauce 130
Meatball noodle soup 80
Meatballs 215
Mexican breakfast hash 56
Mexican chopped salad 191
Mexican spinach casserole 172
Mocha lace biscuits 222
Mug muffin with beef, mushrooms, and cheese 163
Multi-purpose mini loaves with carrots and thyme 97
Mushroom Chips 221
Mussels mariniere 138

O

Orange ginger squash soup 84

P

Paleo sushi 123
Penne with shrimp 140
Peppered shrimp alfredo 132
Pesto egg salad wrap 108
Pesto pizza 111
Pumpkin and chorizo soup 82

R

Radish scramble 50
Raspberry chia pudding 223

Refrigerator pickles 205
Roasted broccoli salad 105
Roasted red pepper and goat cheese dip 94
Roquefort Pear Salad 189
Rosemary garlic eggplant chips 219

S

Saffron cauliflower soup with sumac oil 103
Salmon Cakes 134
Scrambled eggs with smoked salmon 125
Skirt steak avocado salad 196
Spaghetti squash lasagna 170
Spaghetti squash pancakes 52
Spicy Indian chicken stir fry 151
Sunflower butter salmon with onions 128
Sweet and spicy pickled jalapenos 204

T

Taco cups 174
Thai coconut turkey soup 88
Thai pork salad with kelp noodles 187
Twisted tuna salad 126

Z

Zucchini pasta salad 198

www.ingramcontent.com/pod-product-compliance
Lightning Source LLC
Chambersburg PA
CBHW051403070526
44584CB00023B/3269